IF YOUR

CW00376751

JOANNE ELLIOTT
so she has first-hand ex
faced. She is currently writing full-time, but has been a
teacher, social worker, university lecturer, school
director and charity organizer. She was born in New
York, and now lives in Northern Ireland.

Overcoming Common Problems Series

The ABC of Eating
Coping with anorexia, bulimia and
compulsive eating
JOY MELVILLE

Acne
How it's caused and how to cure it
PAUL VAN RIEL

An A–Z of Alternative Medicine
BRENT Q. HAFEN AND KATHRYN J.
FRANDSEN

Arthritis
Is your suffering really necessary?
DR WILLIAM FOX

Birth Over Thirty
SHEILA KITZINGER

Body Language
How to read others' thoughts by their gestures
ALLAN PEASE

Calm Down
How to cope with frustration and anger
DR PAUL HAUCK

Common Childhood Illnesses
DR PATRICIA GILBERT

Coping with Depression and Elation
DR PATRICK McKEON

Curing Arthritis Cookbook
MARGARET HILLS

Curing Arthritis – The Drug-free Way
MARGARET HILLS

Depression
DR PAUL HAUCK

Divorce and Separation
ANGELA WILLANS

Enjoying Motherhood
DR BRUCE PITT

The Epilepsy Handbook
SHELAGH McGOVERN

**Everything You Need to Know about Contact
Lenses**
DR ROBERT YOUNGSON

**Everything You Need to Know about Your
Eyes**
DR ROBERT YOUNGSON

Everything You Need to Know about Shingles
DR ROBERT YOUNGSON

Family First Aid and Emergency Handbook
DR ANDREW STANWAY

Fears and Phobias
What they are and how to overcome them
DR TONY WHITEHEAD

Feverfew
A traditional herbal remedy for migraine and
arthritis
DR STEWART JOHNSON

Fight Your Phobia and Win
DAVID LEWIS

Fit Kit
DAVID LEWIS

Flying Without Fear
TESSA DUCKWORTH AND DAVID
MILLER

Goodbye Backache
DR DAVID IMRIE WITH COLLEEN
DIMSON

Guilt
Why it happens and how to overcome it
DR VERNON COLEMAN

How to Bring Up your Child Successfully
DR PAUL HAUCK

How to Control your Drinking
DRS W. MILLER AND R. MUNOZ

How to Cope with Stress
DR PETER TYRER

Overcoming Common Problems Series

Overcoming Common Problems Series

Overcoming Common Problems

IF YOUR CHILD IS DIABETIC

An answer book for parents

Joanne Elliott

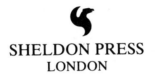

SHELDON PRESS
LONDON

First published in Great Britain in 1987 by
Sheldon Press, SPCK, Marylebone Road, London NW1 4DU

British Library Cataloguing in Publication Data
Elliott, Joanne
  If your child is diabetic: an answer book
  for parents. — (Overcoming common problems)
  1. Diabetes in children — Popular works
  I. Title   II. Series
  618.92′462   RJ420.D5

  ISBN 0–85969–533–6
  ISBN 0–85969–534–4 Pbk

Filmset by Deltatype, Ellesmere Port, Cheshire
Printed in Great Britain by
Richard Clay Ltd, Bungay, Suffolk

Contents

This book is dedicated to the men and women of the British Diabetic Association who give so generously of their time and energy to make life better for diabetics everywhere.

Did you know that . . . .

● Diabetic girls often menstruate later than their non-diabetic sisters.

● Diabetics should eat a low-fat diet.

● Disposable syringes can be re-used.

● Children who cannot eat because of illness need more insulin not less.

● Urine testing equipment is provided on prescription but blood testing equipment is not.

● 'Freezing' the injection site with an ice cube can make injections less painful.

This book provides hundreds of useful facts about childhood diabetes.

Foreword

Most books published to help diabetics are written by doctors who are experts in the medical and scientific aspects of the condition, but they are not actually involved in the day to day management of the diabetic in the home situation.

This book is quite different in that the author is the mother of a young girl who developed insulin dependent diabetes at the age of eight years and is now fourteen. So it is the product of much personal experience of the daily management of a diabetic child and provides the answers to the innumerable questions which parents wish to ask, but are often reluctant to do in a busy out-patient clinic which they attend three or four times a year.

All the questions are relevant, and the answers sensible and easily understood. An important point made is the need of diabetic children to have parents who are interested in their welfare; sophisticated tests will not produce good glucose levels if the child is unhappy.

This book is written clearly and contains much helpful information in compact form without the use of difficult, scientific terms. Its comprehensive content and good advice should make it a trusted reference book, not only at the very upsetting time of initial diagnosis but also throughout the lifetime of the diabetic child.

In my opinion the text is concise, accurate and easy to read. I would commend it wholeheartedly to young diabetics and their families.

S. L. Campbell, M.D., F.R.C.P.I.
Senior Consultant Paediatrician
Diabetic Clinic
Royal Belfast Hospital for Sick Children

Introduction

Recently I was asked to speak to a group of parents whose children had developed diabetes. The topic I was given was 'How parents can help'. Not knowing just how to begin, I asked my young diabetic daughter what she thought was the best way for parents to help a diabetic child. Her answer was short and simple. 'Parents can help', she declared, 'by knowing everything'.

No one can know everything about diabetes. There is so much which has yet to be discovered. We, as parents, though, can certainly make a start; for we start with the knowledge that the more we learn about this disease, the better we can control it.

I am a parent like you; the training I have had in diabetes has been on-the-job training, learning to cope with my child's daily life. You are learning now in the same way that I did. This learning process is painful. Many aspects of diabetes are frightening. No one wants to think about the complications which could arise in later life. Refusing to think about them, however, will not make them go away. On the contrary, learning to control this disease more effectively will reduce the possibility that your child will develop complications.

Learning does more than promote better diabetic control. It also promotes better mental health. When a child is first diagnosed, it is a bitter blow. 'Why me?' asks the child. 'Why my child?' ask the parents; fear, guilt and despair hold them fast.

The child is frightened to be different. The parents fear that they cannot cope with the demands that this condition will require. They feel depressed and helpless in the face of this unseen menace which has reached out from nowhere to threaten their family. By mastering this fear and pain, by learning to control the disease instead of being controlled by it, parents learn to fight back. *It is a fight which can be won.*

The fact that you, the parent, are sitting here reading this book

3

instead of collapsing into bed with 'nerves' or emptying a bottle of spirits in the local pub means that you have already taken the first step. You have decided that you are not helpless. You and your child will learn. You will adjust. You will fight back and your life will be normal again. It is my aim to give you the necessary weapons so that you will win.

In my work as a volunteer diabetic educator and through my contacts with the British Diabetic Association, I have spoken to hundreds of parents. We have discussed our mutual problems by the hour. As parents together we talked about the things that we were too diffident to mention to the doctor or the nurse. We talked about the moodiness of the diabetic child, about his fear of being 'different'. We talked about our dread of night-time hypos, about school and exam pressures, about difficult grandparents and well-meaning but thoughtless friends. Learning to cope with these problems is as important to your child's health as learning good injection techniques and counting carbohydrates. For your child is, first of all, himself, not merely a 'diabetic'.

In this book, I try to cover all aspects of diabetic care, physical and emotional, to supply as many answers as I can to the endless stream of questions that you, the parent, need to ask.

1

About Diabetes

Q. What exactly is diabetes?

A. Diabetes, or diabetes mellitus (sugar diabetes) is a disorder of the means by which the body changes the food we eat into energy. It occurs when the pancreas, a gland which lies behind the stomach stops making enough insulin. If too little insulin is produced by the pancreas, too much of the sugar called glucose gathers in the blood. Eventually the glucose is carrying with it large amounts of water. The early symptom of diabetes is frequent passing of urine which in turn causes great thirst. In addition, without insulin the body cannot store reserves of glucose, protein and fat and so rapid weight loss follows. Without insulin treatment, dehydration, coma and eventually death will result.

Q. Why does this happen?

A. The precise cause is unknown. The body appears to destroy its own insulin-producing cells by substances called antibodies. The tendency to produce these antibodies may be inherited. Not everyone, though, who is predisposed to the disease will develop it. It is possible that another factor, possibly a virus, may be necessary to trigger the production of these antibodies in a person with an inherited tendency to diabetes.

Q. Could I have known that my child had such a tendency?

A. No, at present there is no way that you could have known this. In the future, perhaps, there will be a way of identifying children at risk.

Q. If I had brought my child to the doctor earlier, could the diabetes have been prevented?

A. No. The earlier the condition is diagnosed, the less marked will be the symptoms but the disease would still exist even if diagnosed on the first day.

Q. Is there anything that I could have done to keep my child from becoming diabetic?
A. No, nothing. The ability of the pancreas to produce insulin is probably diminished for many years before the person actually becomes diabetic. People with an inherited tendency towards diabetes produce substances called islet cell antibodies. These antibodies destroy the insulin-producing cells. This process begins a long time before there are any symptoms of diabetes. It may even occur at birth.

Q. Did I do anything to contribute to it? If I had fed him differently, perhaps prevented him from eating so many sweets, would I have been able to prevent it?
A. Nothing you did or failed to do has had the slightest effect on the fact that your child developed diabetes. Blaming yourself is very natural but completely unjustified.

Q. Will he outgrow it?
A. I wish I could tell you that he would, but unfortunately, it isn't true. He will always be diabetic. I was plagued, in the first few years after my child became diabetic, by well-meaning friends who assured me that she would outgrow it. It is not possible.

Q. At what age can children develop diabetes?
A. At any age. Most children who develop diabetes do so during the school years but it can, however, develop much earlier. Although rare, it can happen in infancy.

Q. Can diabetes be prevented?
A. Recently, much work has been done to identify children at risk with a view towards prevention. This work is still in the early stages. In the future, however, it might be possible to prevent the development of diabetes in a susceptible person.

Q. Is diabetes difficult to diagnose?
A. No, the symptoms of insulin dependent diabetes are marked, making diagnosis easy.

Q. What are the symptoms?
A. Excessive passing of urine, thirst, weight loss, fatigue.

Q. My child had these symptoms for a long time before my doctor suggested that it might be diabetes. Why did this happen?
A. Diabetes in children is not common. In the United Kingdom and Ireland, only one child in 600 under sixteen is diabetic It is unlikely that your family doctor has had many such cases.

Q. Now that my child has been diagnosed, shall I continue to take him to my family doctor or shall I take him to a special diabetic clinic?
A. Unless your family doctor is extremely interested in diabetes, has the means of using hospital laboratory facilities for quarterly blood tests, and keeps up to date with the latest development in diabetic care and research, it is better to attend a specialist clinic.

Q. Where are these clinics located?
A. Your family doctor can refer you to one near your home. Most hospitals have such clinics.

Q. What can the diabetic clinic offer my child that my family doctor cannot?
A. The diabetic clinic will, undoubtedly, be staffed by one or more consultants who have a special interest in diabetes. They will have the experience of treating hundreds, perhaps thousands of diabetics. They will have access to the latest equipment which is being developed constantly. They will have books and magazines which you may be able to borrow. Some clinics have video films and colour slides as well. Some even have teaching programmes about diabetes for home computers. The diabetic clinic is a place for learning for you as well as your child. In addition to its educational facilities,

the clinic's staff will include a dietician. Some have child psychologists, eye specialists, nurse specialists in diabetes and other trained persons whose job it is to help diabetics. The clinic will have laboratory facilities and be connected to eye, heart and kidney units to detect and treat possible complications before they become severe. Many clinics maintain close relations with self-help groups like the ones run by the British Diabetic Association. These groups can provide much assistance.

Q. Do these clinics treat diabetics of all ages or do they specialize?

A. Most clinics treat diabetics of all ages, but in large cities you can generally find paediatric diabetic clinics for children only. If you live in or near a large city, this is the kind of care to seek. The paediatric diabetic clinic is a very specialized place where the emphasis is on reassurance. The waiting rooms are filled with toys; the nurses are skilled at taking blood from small veins; the doctors are specially trained to deal sympathetically with anxious parents.

Q. If I take my child to a special diabetic clinic, will my family doctor be kept informed of his progress?

A. Regular letters will be sent to your family doctor to keep him up to date. It is your family doctor, too, who will write the prescriptions for your child's diabetic needs.

Q. My family doctor looks after elderly people who are diabetic. Why don't they attend a special diabetic clinic?

A. Diabetes in the middle-aged and elderly is common in our culture. The doctor in general practice probably has many such patients.

Q. I have several elderly relatives who are diabetic. Could my child have inherited the diabetes from them?

A. It is unlikely that your child's diabetes was inherited directly from these relatives. Diabetes in this older age group is called Type 2 Diabetes or Non-insulin Dependent Diabetes.

It is different from the diabetes that your child has developed which is called Type 1 Diabetes or Insulin Dependent Diabetes.

Q. What is the difference?
A. In Type 2 Diabetes, the pancreas is less active than normal but it is still capable of producing insulin. If its function is assisted by weight loss, special diet and exercise, often adequate insulin production returns. If it does not, the pancreas can be stimulated chemically to produce more insulin.

Q. If my child were to be put on a special diet would he be able to make more insulin?
A. Even on a special diet, his natural insulin would not be sufficient.

Q. What about stimulating the pancreas chemically? Does this mean taking tablets?
A. It does, but these tablets are only suitable for those diabetics who are capable of producing adequate amounts of natural insulin. Your child's pancreas is unable to do this. The small amount of natural insulin that he may be making at the time of diagnosis will be reduced further in time. He needs insulin by injection to supplement his inadequate supply.

Q. Why can't insulin be given by mouth?
A. The digestive system would destroy it before it could be used.

Q. Couldn't the tablet be coated with something that the body won't destroy?
A. This is a possibility for the future, but at present, no one has been able to make such a tablet. There is, however, a great deal of research going on all the time in many countries all over the world. Better products will be available in years to come. A cure could lie right around the corner; no one knows. Diabetic research takes place in many countries around the world.

Q. Is diabetes a dangerous disease?

A. Once the condition is diagnosed and insulin therapy begun, the diabetes can be brought under control. It can do hidden damage, though. This hidden damage can lead to other diseases in later life which are serious. Diabetes can damage the small blood vessels. Such damage can cause the development of heart, kidney, eye and nerve disease and poor blood supply to the feet. With good control, however, the likelihood of your child developing any of these complications in later life is reduced. That is why your knowledge of diabetic control is important.

Q. Will it get worse?

A. In the beginning, the pancreas is still producing some insulin. As soon as treatment begins, the pancreas may recover some of its ability to produce insulin. The amount that has to be added by injection is small, so small that you may begin to wonder if the doctor has made a mistake; perhaps your child is not diabetic after all. But after a time more pancreatic cells will die and the amount of natural insulin will diminish. He will need more by injection. The early period when the pancreas is still functioning fairly well is called the Honeymoon Period.

Q. How long does the Honeymoon Period last?

A. It varies from a few months to a year or more. There is some evidence to suggest that the Honeymoon Period can be prolonged by good control.

Q. If insulin production is improved during the Honeymoon Period, will a child be able to stop his injections?

A. It is very rare for enough pancreatic function to return for injections to stop altogether.

Q. How can I learn more about diabetes?

A. Read all you can on the subject. A reading list is given at the end of the book. Also, join the British Diabetic Association. The BDA is a non-profit charity devoted to the welfare of diabetics. They produce books, pamphlets, films, scientific journals and an excellent magazine called *Balance* which comes out six times a year. *Balance* is sent free of charge to members. It contains articles about diabetic care, new research, letters from readers, problems and advice, recipes, stories and games for children. It is a treasure-house of information about diabetes. Reading it regularly will keep you in touch with new products designed to make life easier as well as with the latest developments in science. You will also benefit from the knowledge that you are not alone. Other diabetics and their families have similar problems. Learning how they solved them will make yours less difficult. Membership in the BDA is £5 a year. People on Supplementary Benefit pay £1. Children under sixteen may join free for one year.

Q. How do I join?
A. Many commonly used diabetic products contain application forms in the packaging. If you haven't come across any forms, write to the British Diabetic Association, 10 Queen Anne Street, London, W1M 0BD. Give them your child's name, address and age. You'll find that it is the single most worthwhile effort you can make to help the entire family in this very difficult situation.

Q. Are there local self-help groups that I can join?
A. The BDA has branches and Parents' Groups everywhere in the UK. If you would like to join one, ask for the name of the Secretary in your diabetic clinic. If you cannot get the information there, write to the BDA and ask them to refer you to a group in your area.

Q. What do these groups do?
A. They provide a forum for learning about diabetes by arranging meetings with interesting speakers, having discussion groups, raising money for diabetic research, having parties and social events for members, especially children. Some provide equipment free or at a discount to members. By joining with others to achieve a common goal, many people find that they are better able to cope with stress.

Q. Can diabetics in the Irish Republic join the BDA?
A. Yes.

Q. What else does the BDA do?
A. Through its many publications and films, the BDA can keep you and your family up to date on developments of interest.

Q. Won't our family doctor be aware of new developments in diabetes through the medical journals?
A. It is unrealistic to expect your family doctor, who has a very small number of diabetic patients in his practice, to keep up completely with the news in so specialized a subject.

2

Insulin and Injections

Q. Where does insulin come from?
A. Until recently, all insulin for medical use was made from cow and pig pancreases. Now a synthetic insulin has been developed. This synthetic insulin is identical to human insulin. It is also free from many impurities which sometimes provoked allergic reactions in the past.

Q. How is synthetic human insulin made?
A. There are two methods of making it at the moment. One is by making a small adjustment to purified pig insulin to get it to correspond exactly to natural human insulin. The other method is by programming certain bacteria to manufacture it through genetic engineering techniques. It is quite an important advance because it means that the manufacture of insulin is no longer dependent on the availability of animal pancreases.

Q. Does this insulin have a special name?
A. It is called Human Insulin.

Q. Is that different from U100?
A. U100 refers to the strength of the insulin. Until 1984, diabetics in the United Kingdom and the Republic of Ireland were using insulin of varying strengths. Forty and eighty strengths were the most common although some diabetics were using twenty strength insulin. Now, everyone has been switched to a single strength called U100.

Q. Why was this done?
A. It was done to eliminate dosage errors and to bring diabetics in the UK and Ireland into line with the practice in the US, Canada and Australia.

Q. Will my child be on the new strength of insulin?
A. Yes.

Q. Will he be on an animal insulin or a human one?

A. The doctor in hospital will prescribe the type of insulin which he thinks best for your child. All modern insulins are purified and the results are generally good. Studies of comparative insulins have shown no difference between control on animal and human insulins.

Q. Does insulin have to be kept in the refrigerator?

A. It should be kept cool. A fridge is best but if you have no fridge, a cool place in the kitchen where meat or milk would be kept fresh will do. It must never be allowed to freeze. Keep it out of the deep freeze, and don't put it directly under the ice-making compartment of the fridge. While travelling by air, too, it is important to keep the insulin with you in the cabin of the plane. Do not allow it to be placed in the baggage compartment where it might be subjected to extremely low temperatures.

Q. Should it be warmed before injection?

A. Very cold insulin injected into a warm body is uncomfortable. It is better to warm it slightly before injecting. This can be done easily by rubbing the bottles between your hands for a minute or two before filling the syringe. Most diabetics store extra bottles of insulin in the fridge but keep the bottle or bottles in current use at room temperature to eliminate this problem.

Q. My child was given two different bottles of insulin, one clear and one cloudy. What is the difference between them?

A. The clear insulin is a quick-acting variety. The cloudy insulin takes longer to act. It contains other substances which slow down its activity.

Q. Why does he need both kinds?

A. The quick-acting is useful to provide cover for the meal which comes soon after injection time. The cloudy is useful for a meal which may come several hours later. Insulin is required over a 24-hour period. A mixture of clear and cloudy insulins helps to reduce the body's natural insulin release pattern.

Q. How soon after injection does the insulin begin to work?

A. Clear insulin starts to lower the blood glucose in half-an-hour. It has its strongest effect three to four hours later. It stops working about eight hours after injection. Insulin injected at 7.30am will work at breakfast time (8.00am). Its peak action will be between 11.00am and noon. It will run out by 4.00pm.

Cloudy insulin works more slowly. It has its strongest effect eight to fourteen hours after injection. Cloudy insulin taken before breakfast (7.30am) will be acting at the time of the evening meal (6.00pm). Cloudy insulin taken before the evening meal (6.00pm), will cover breakfast the next morning.

Q. Why are some children on one injection a day, some on two?

A. Sometimes young children are started on one injection a day. This is usually a mixture of clear and cloudy. The clear insulin covers breakfast, mid-morning snack, lunch and mid-afternoon snack. The cloudy covers the evening meal and a before-bedtime snack. Young children go to bed early and usually don't require food during the night. This regime is appropriate for them. Also, it is likely that the young child, having recently become diabetic, is still making some natural insulin. This amount is insufficient for his needs, but when supplemented with a single daily injection, can often be adequate for normal health and growth.

Some children, however, are started on two injections daily even though they are very young. Some doctors think that since most diabetics will have to change to two injections eventually, it is easier to begin this routine in the early years.

Q. Which is better, a one injection routine or two?

A. There are advantages and disadvantages to both. One obvious advantage to a one injection routine is that injections always appear to be the biggest problem in the beginning and this routine reduces the number of injections by half. A disadvantage is that the child is tied to an early evening meal time. On a one injection routine, he must have his evening meal when his cloudy insulin taken in the morning is acting strongly. If the injection was taken at 7.30 in the morning, he must eat by 5 o'clock or his blood glucose will drop too low. While a three-year-old is happy to eat at 5 o'clock, a school-age child may prefer to be out playing with his friends at that time.

If your doctor has strong reasons for recommending a particular regime, I suggest that you follow his recommendation. Some children have more natural insulin production than others in the early days after diagnosis, and your doctor's choice of routine may be influenced by that factor. If your doctor puts your child on a two-injection routine from the beginning, you can console yourself (and the child), with the thought that eventually he would have to change to that routine anyway, and that the two-injection routine allows more latitude.

Q. If he is on two injections a day, can the evening meal be eaten at any time?

A. It is important to stick to a fairly regular timetable for meals and injections in order to ensure that the insulin in circulation is the right amount at the time. You need to be certain that meals are taken when the insulin is at its peak action so that the blood glucose does not fall below normal. It is possible, however, to be more flexible on a two-injection routine, moving the evening meal time to 6.00pm or 7.00pm without problems. On a two-injection routine, the morning dose of cloudy insulin is smaller than it would be on a single dose regime. The afternoon snack can be taken after school, allowing more freedom in the early evening for play before the second injection is taken, half-an-hour before the evening meal. In fact, if your child is on a one-injection routine and needs to change to two injections a day, this can be a convincing argument. If he were willing to take two injections, he would not be tied to an early evening meal and would be spared the risk of low blood glucose around 5 o'clock, when he might want to be playing football or riding his bicycle.

Q. You say that injections appear to be the biggest problem at first. Do they get easier after a while?

A. It is hard to believe when your child is first diagnosed, but injections really do get easier after a while. In a year or two, injections will become almost automatic. Your child will hardly mind them as much as brushing his teeth. I know that this statement sounds unbelievable to a parent of a newly diagnosed child, but it really is true. After a while, the child will become completely casual about injections and regard anyone who balks at them as foolish. (I don't guarantee, however, that parents will feel the same way!)

Q. If my child has to take both clear and cloudy insulin once or twice a day, does this mean that he has to take two injections each time, or can the two types be mixed in the same syringe?

A. It is usual to mix both insulins in the same syringe. You do it in the following way:

1 Wash your hands.
2 Clean the tops of the bottles with industrial spirit.
3 Shake the bottle of cloudy insulin to ensure that it is mixed.
4 With your syringe, inject air into the cloudy insulin in an amount corresponding to the prescribed units of insulin. (If you need to draw up 10 units of insulin, inject 10 units of air.)
5 Withdraw the syringe. Do not draw up any insulin yet.
6 Insert the same syringe into the clear insulin. Inject the required units of air. (If you need to withdraw 15 units of insulin, inject 15 units of air.)
7 Do not remove the syringe. Draw up the clear insulin.
8 Return to the cloudy bottle. Draw up the cloudy insulin.
9 Tap out any bubbles which may have appeared in the syringe.

Q. Why is it necessary to clean the tops of the bottles with spirit?

A. I recommend cleaning the bottle tops only because it is likely that your child will keep his diabetic kit in a plastic box which soon will become a repository for crumbs, used syringes, plastic testing strips, sweet papers, notebook, pencils, etc. It will probably make you feel better to introduce a hygienic note.

Q. I have asked for spirit at my local chemist and have been given surgical spirit. Is this different from the industrial spirit you mention?

A. Surgical spirit is oily and leaves a film. Industrial spirit is better, although it is more difficult to obtain. All chemists, however, can supply little cotton swabs which are impregnated with industrial spirit. These swabs are very handy. They come on a roll. Each swab is individually wrapped in paper. You use them once and throw them away. The most common brand is called Medi-Swabs. They are available on prescription.

Q. Would industrial spirit on a piece of cotton wool do?

A. It will, of course. This cleaning process is not terribly important and can be omitted. If you are on holiday and find that you have run out of Medi-Swabs or spirit and cotton wool, don't panic. It is extremely unlikely that bacteria will find their way from the top of the insulin bottle into the syringe.

Q. What do you do if, in the middle of filling the syringe, you find that you have made a mistake?

A. Discard the insulin and start again. Soon you and your child will become expert and mistakes will be rare. In the beginning, everyone is clumsy and uncertain about injections. Expertise is quickly acquired. Before long, you will be helping someone new.

Q. Is there any way that I can make injections less painful for my child? He gets upset each time. This is upsetting to me too.

A. You might try putting an ice cube on the site for a short time, to make the skin less sensitive. He might think it fun. In fact, many children like to suck ice cubes and you might let him do that after he has chilled the site, to distract him from the actual injection.

Most of the unpleasantness associated with injections is psychological. The prick of the needle is almost painless if the needle is sharp and fine. Some needle brands are lubricated for greater comfort. Much of the 'pain' is actually fear, his and yours. Children can sense fear much as animals can. If you try to present a calm and reassuring front to your child at injection time, it will help him to relax. If this is difficult for you, you might find that another family member, perhaps an older child, can help. It does not always have to be Mummy or Daddy who do these things. Don't feel that you have failed if you withdraw in favour of Granny or sister. A child newly diagnosed can present many problems. It often takes the resources of the entire family to cope. Just keep telling yourself that this trying time will not last forever.

Q. Is it more painful to take a long time over the injection, or to do it quickly? My child accepted injections in hospital when they were given by the nurses but whinges when I do them. I am inexperienced, of course, and slow.

A. The least painful injection is the one which is given quickest. The nerve endings are in the skin. The quicker you can penetrate the layers of skin, the less pain is felt.

Q. How can I increase my speed?

A. Speed will come automatically with experience. Have you ever watched a master chef on TV cutting an onion? How deftly he dissects it into hundreds of tiny even pieces! It takes years of practice, however, to develop this quick, apparently careless ease. One idea which might help you is to practise with a chicken. Next time you cook a chicken, try piercing its flesh with an insulin syringe. Note how much easier it is to get through the skin quickly if you hold it firmly and toss the needle in like a dart.

Q. What do you do about air bubbles in the syringe? I am terrified about injecting air into a vein and killing my child.

A. This is one of the most common fears that everyone has about giving injections to himself or to anyone else. If you look at an insulin syringe, though, you will notice that it is quite narrow and that the needle is short. The places where you are injecting insulin have layers of fat under the skin. The small needle cannot each the large blood vessels. It can only go into the fat layers. Also, if you look at the air bubbles which appear in the syringe, they are tiny. There isn't room for large bubbles of air inside such a narrow space. Such small quantities of air will not do any harm.

If you cannot get rid of the bubbles by flicking the syringe with your finger, turn it upside down after it is filled. Wait until the contents settle, and turn it up again. You will find that the insulin has returned to the front of the syringe, leaving the air bubbles behind. Inject before the bubbles make their way down.

Q. What do you do if some insulin oozes out again?
A. This only happens occasionally. If it happens to you, quickly pull the skin to one side, closing off the puncture. Next time you inject, pull the skin aside before injection. As soon as the syringe is empty and the needle withdrawn, return the skin to its original position, thus closing the hole and preventing leakage.

Q. Should there be a little lump under the skin after injection?
A. No. If you are getting a lump, the injection is too shallow. Make certain that you are putting the needle straight down at a right angle to the skin.

Q. Why is there a small amount of bleeding sometimes?
A. You have probably punctured a very tiny blood vessel called a capillary. This is nothing to worry about. The bleeding will stop in seconds. It may discolour the skin for a few days. This happens to everyone sometimes, but it is not a frequent occurrence. Don't worry about it.

Q. Is there a danger of injecting into a large blood vessel?
A. If you use the sites recommended by the doctor (see illustration on p 109), there is no danger. These sites have

been chosen because they do not contain major blood vessels or nerves.

Q. How important is it to vary the sites? My child is resistant to the idea of injecting anywhere but one small area of leg.

A. It is quite important. If one site were used repeatedly, the tissue may become hard and insulin absorption irregular. Control will suffer. Other problems may arise as a result. The favourite site may become pain resistant, which will make the child favour it even more. Avoid this situation from the beginning. It can lead to trouble. Make sure that your child understands the reasons for changing the sites. If he is young, perhaps you could make a little chart together to hang in his room, showing the correct sites and labelling them 'Monday', 'Tuesday', etc. You could enlarge the illustration in Appendix 1. If he is willing to inject into his tummy as well as the leg (arms are generally too small in young children), let him do the morning injection into his tummy every day, and the evening one into his leg, or vice versa. This sort of regularity gives the best results because the insulin is absorbed at the same rate at the same time every day. The first principle of good control is *regularity*.

Q. Are there any other factors which affect the rate of absorption of insulin?

A. Insulin is most quickly absorbed from the abdomen, then the arms, followed by the thighs and buttocks. Heat and activity affect it as well. Heat causes insulin to circulate more rapidly through the bloodstream. If the insulin injection is followed by a hot bath or a long, hot shower, the circulation is speeded up. Blood glucose levels are lowered quickly.

If vigorous exercise like cycling follows an injection into the thighs or legs, the insulin circulates more quickly than it would if the diabetic were still. This is a useful characteristic of insulin which you can manipulate to increase control. For example, if a blood test were done before an injection which shows the blood glucose to be high, rather than increase the dose of clear insulin and thus possible risk of hypo a few hours later, it is possible to reduce the glucose level by increasing the circulation of the insulin.

Q. Is there any other way in which this can be done other than by hot water?

A. You could rub the spot gently for five minutes, raising the skin temperature by friction, or you could warm it by placing a hot water bottle wrapped in a towel on the site.

Q. Should parents insist that the injection sites be varied?

A. Suggestion is better than insistence. A tactful way to get your child to vary the sites is to send him to one of the children's holiday camps run by the British Diabetic Association. There he will see other children injecting into their arms and tummies as well as their legs. He will want to try it too. Children are natural conformists. They are happiest doing what other children are doing. It gives them a sense of belonging. These camps are priced within everyone's budget. In Great Britain, the BDA will apply for a local authority grant for any family who needs one. In Northern Ireland, local BDA branches will sponsor any diabetic child, member or non-member, who wants to attend. These camps are extremely valuable especially for the child who is newly diagnosed.

Q. What sort of activities do they have at the camp?

A. All the usual holiday activities are catered for. There is swimming, hiking, perhaps cycling or pony-trekking, canoeing, art and crafts, discos, all sports, etc. The children are supervised by trained staff, medical and non-medical. The meals are prepared by dieticians. Your child can enjoy himself in complete security and learn about his diabetes at the same time. The camps also give parents a week off from the responsibility of caring for a child with special needs, which can be very difficult at first.

Q. How can I find out more about these camps?

A. Ask in your diabetic clinic, your local BDA branch or Parents' Group, or write to Youth Department, British

Diabetic Association, 10, Queen Anne Street, London, W1M 0BD.

Q. Is injection the only way of taking insulin?

A. At the moment, it is the only method in general use. Research is going on every day, however, to find better methods of insulin delivery.

One of these new methods is the insulin pump. This is a device worn outside the body, perhaps on a belt at the waist or in a shoulder holster. The insulin pump contains a small reservoir of insulin connected to a plastic tube. A fine needle is attached which is inserted under the skin, usually at the tummy. The pump releases a small quantity of insulin every few seconds. A larger dose can be released at meal times. Some pumps have a manual release for the mealtime insulin, allowing the person to eat at any time he chooses, or even to skip meals. Some pumps release this insulin at predetermined times during the day.

One interesting new device looks like a pen. It is designed to be worn in the pocket of a jacket or school blazer. The 'pen' makes subcutaneous injections more convenient, so insulin can be given before each meal fairly easily. When insulin is required for a meal, a button is pressed on the top of the pen which releases 2 units of clear insulin at a time. The wearer presses the button as many times as is necessary to get his required dose. On this regime, the diabetic must also take a single injection of long-acting insulin daily. It is useful for business people and students whose meal times may occasionally be erratic.

Scientists are also working on a device which can be implanted into the body like a cardiac pacemaker. This pump would be able to be filled with insulin from outside of the body via a needle. Its reservoir would be large enough, however, so that it wouldn't have to be topped up very often. This implantable pump is still experimental. There are many technical problems which still have to be solved.

Q. Are these pumps suitable for children?

A. Pumps are very exciting and most parents see them as a way to get away from injections, always a problem in the first few months after diagnosis. They may not, however, be the answer for everyone. At the moment, the smallest pump in use is still larger than a cigarette box. Most are quite a bit larger. The needle which connects it to the body must be moved every few days to avoid infection at the site. To ensure that the pump is working properly the wearer must test his blood 5 or 6 times a day. Many children would find this irksome. The pump has to be removed for swimming and bathing and care taken that air does not get into the plastic tubing. It may have to be removed for other active games as well. I know children who have pumps and who are doing very well on them.

It is not the answer for all, though. Certainly, wearing a pump is a big commitment for a child and one not to be undertaken lightly. The child must know quite a bit about how to control his diabetes before he is able to handle a pump. He must be motivated to perform constant blood tests. He must accept the restrictions on dress. If the tube is to pass from a device worn outside the clothes to under the clothes, holes must be made. Fashion must take second place. There can be other problems as well.

Q. What other problems might arise?

A. Sometimes needles clog and the insulin cannot get through the tube. Blood glucose may rise very quickly in this situation. Infections at the site are frequent and some children have to change the needle every day in order to avoid them. Still, for those children who tolerate the pump well, control can be excellent.

Q. Would you recommend a pump for children?

A. Pump therapy is new. I think that parents should be patient and wait until research and development is more advanced. It is hoped that, eventually, the pump would be able to be linked to a blood glucose sensor which would test the glucose levels and automatically release the correct amount of insulin. This would be virtually an artificial pancreas. If such a device could be developed, it would revolutionize the treatment of diabetes.

Q. It is likely that such a device will be developed?
A. Much work is being done in this country and abroad to develop such a pump. With the recent gigantic advances in microtechnology, I think that it is a distinct possibility and offers much hope for the future.

Q. Are there any diabetics in the UK or the Republic of Ireland wearing pumps at the moment?
A. Yes, some diabetics are wearing them and the number will increase in the future. Problems which arose with earlier pumps are being solved and this form of insulin delivery is improving all the time. It is still too early, however, to know whether the pump is the answer for all.

Q. Are any of these pump users children?
A. Yes, some of them are. If you would like to talk to someone who is wearing a pump or who is the parent of a child wearing a pump, your diabetic clinic should be able to arrange it.

Q. Are there any other new devices which are suitable for children?
A. One interesting device is called the Infusor Button. It is a flat plastic device about the size of coin. A plastic tube leads to a fine needle which is inserted into the tummy and the button is taped into place. At injection time, the user injects into the button rather than into his body. The injection therefore is painless. It enables the user to inject many times during the day rather than once or twice. He can take clear insulin whenever he eats, mimicking more precisely the natural insulin release of the non-diabetic. He can also take an injection of a long acting insulin to give a small amount of insulin over a 24-hour period. For the conscientious user, the button can mean better control.

Q. Would it be suitable for children?

A. Perhaps for the older child. To get the maximum advantage from the button, frequent blood tests would have to be done. Also, the button itself would have to be moved fairly frequently to avoid infections at the site. The manufacturers recommend moving it every three days. This, however, is very much an individual reaction. Some people might require more frequent moves. It is certainly an interesting idea, though, and one which may become popular. It is also inexpensive.

Q. Where are these devices sold?

A. Many are advertised for sale through the journals and publications of the British Diabetic Association. They are also sold by medical mail order houses. Your diabetic clinic might have literature describing them. If not, they can tell you where to find such literature. All these devices, however, require a high level of interest and knowledge. For the child who is newly diagnosed, there is no reasonable substitute for injections.

Q. Is there any other research at the moment which might eliminate the need for injections?

A. There is an exciting line of research going on in America. Scientists are trying to transplant insulin-producing cells from a healthy pancreas into a diabetic. Previous attempts to do this have failed because the new cells were quickly attacked by the body's immune system. Now, a way is being looked at to wrap the cells in a special membrane which will prevent destructive antibodies from reaching the cells yet allow the passage of insulin out and the passage of nutrients and glucose in to keep the cells alive. The cells would be placed in the body of the diabetic by an annual injection.

This technique is being tried out on animals at the moment and will go into clinical trials on humans in 1988. There is certainly hope for the future. Never despair. In the last five years enormous advances have been made and most of the new devices which are available to your child today were unknown five years ago. Five years from now, I expect that many, many more will have been developed.

Q. *At the moment, is there any alternative to injections other than pumps.*

A. No.

Q. *Since my child has to have injections, how can I get him to accept them more easily?*

A. The young child has already established a pattern of accepting whatever his parents present to him. If the parents have a matter-of-fact attitude towards injections, he will learn very quickly to accept them. With an older child it may take longer, but, in my experience, children accept injections more readily than their parents would have believed possible. Sometimes play can help. I know one nine year old who played 'hospital' constantly after she was diagnosed. By injecting dolls and teddies she was able to work out her anger at being diabetic. Play like this can be a useful tool and should not be discouraged even if it appears morbid to outsiders. Sometimes, injection aids can be used to get a child 'over the hump'.

Q. *What are injection aids?*

A. These are devices which some children find make injections easier. There are two on the market at the moment, the Palmer Injector Gun and the Hypoguard Painless Injector. The Gun is fitted with a filled syringe and placed on the injection site. The trigger is pulled; the syringe surges forward and the needle enters very quickly. The plunger is then pushed in manually. The Painless Injector is a stainless steel cylinder which is fitted over the end of the syringe hiding the needle. The cylinder is placed on the site, given a push and the needle shoots in quickly. The plunger is pressed manually.

Q. *Where can I get these aids?*

A. They are advertised regularly in *Balance*, the magazine of the British Diabetic Association. You can buy them by mail order.

Q. *Are these aids a good idea?*

A. They have certain advantages. Using the Painless Injector, for example, the needle enters the body at the correct angle, lessening the chance of bruising. The psychological effect of screening the needle from view helps the squeamish. There are disadvantages too. Often, a child becomes so dependent on the aid that he will not inject without it. This could be a problem if the aid is lost or damaged. I think that if a child is not unduly frightened by injections, it is better for him to learn good injection technique from the beginning. If, however, injections are a trial, if tears and fussing a daily ritual, an injection aid might solve the problem.

Q. *What constitutes good injection technique?*

A. The syringe must be filled correctly (see page 17) and any air bubbles tapped out. A suitable site must be selected (see illustration on p 109) and the child should sit comfortably with his feet on the floor. He should then inject straight in at a right angle to the skin. There is no need to wipe the skin with spirit before taking an insulin injection.

Q. *The nurse in the ward showed us how to inject. She said to inject at an angle of 45 degrees. Which is correct?*

A. If you are using the newest, finest needle available to you (which is the one which will cause the least discomfort) you will find that this needle is only ½ inch long. The nurse in the ward was probably trained at a time when the needles for insulin injections were much longer. If you inject at an angle of 45 degrees with a half inch needle you will get a shallow injection which will leave the insulin in a mass under the skin because it will not reach the subcutaneous layer of fat which lies underneath. Your absorption will be poor and irregular and control will not be at its best. Why not get a new insulin syringe and show it to the nurse? Perhaps she will change her advice.

INSULIN AND INJECTIONS

Q. *I did not know that there were needles of various lengths. Which is the best?*

A. The shortest, finest needles are the most comfortable to use. At the moment, a 28 gauge needle has just come on the market which is lubricated to give an easier injection. The figure 28 refers to the width of the needle. The finer the needle, the higher the number. Look for the shortest needle with the highest gauge number.

Q. *Where can I get these needles?*

A. Your chemist will be able to order them for you. Some people are using needles which are much larger and longer than they need be because their chemist doesn't stock any others. All the needle manufacturers make needles in various sizes. If your chemist asks his manufacturer's representative, he will be able to get them.

Q. *Are there new needles available under the National Health Service?*

A. The National Health Service does not stipulate the size of insulin needles which are on the Drug Tariff. If you are entitled to free needles, you can get them in any size you like.

Q. *Are diabetics entitled to free needles?*

A. Yes. See Appendix 5 for a list of products available under the National Health Service at the time of publication.

Q. *I have seen syringes with the needles attached and some where the needles can be detached. Which are the best?*

A. Many people prefer the disposable syringes with the needles attached because there is no danger of the needle coming off during injecting which can be upsetting. There is really very little difference between them, however. It is slightly more economical to use the disposable syringe with the detachable needles because you can change the needle frequently while re-using the syringe.

Q. *Is it possible to re-use the disposable syringe? The packet warns you to throw them away after one use.*

A. Recent medical surveys have found no incidence of infection due to the re-use of plastic syringes and most doctors advise their patients to use them until the needle is blunt.

Q. *Are disposable needles available under the National Health Service?*

A. In Great Britain, children under 16 who are attending a diabetic clinic in a hospital which has a dispensary, can be dispensed disposable needles. The situation is different in Northern Ireland. I believe that all diabetics in the Irish Republic can receive free disposable syringes. Ask in your clinic. If you find that your child is not entitled to receive disposable syringes under the National Health Service, you can buy a packet of the sort where the needles are detachable and get a good supply of disposable needles for them. You can throw away the needles whenever they get blunt and re-use the syringes until they get sticky or the numbers rub off. It is possible, with care, to make one packet of 10 (which costs just over £1) last for months.

Q. *Is it better to use glass or disposable plastic syringes?*

A. It is probably better to use both, and indeed, as many types of equipment as possible. Children tend to cling to the familiar. The child who has recently become diabetic will, naturally, be anxious. Anxiety will exaggerate the clinging. If he starts out using only one type of syringe, he may become resistant to changing it even if a more suitable type appears on the scene. If he is accustomed, from the beginning, to trying out a variety of equipment, he is less likely to be difficult in this area. Some people use glass syringes for home use and disposables for travelling and for meals out. On the whole, although disposable syringes are not prescribable for all diabetics, the fact that they don't have to be sterilised makes them more convenient. If you re-use them (for a week) a packet costing just over £1 will last for two and a half months.

Q. *If it isn't necessary to sterilise them, what do you do?*

A. After use, replace the plastic cap which fits over the needle. Slide it down over the needle very carefully so that the point of the needle never comes into contact with the plastic (constant contact with a hard surface will blunt the needle). Then store it in a convenient place. A glass on the door of the fridge is often a handy place to store the syringe. It may be kept anywhere, though. My child keeps all her gear in a plastic Tupperware box and an extra set in a handbag for travelling. If she is going out for a meal straight from school, she can just take the little bag with her in the morning and not have to bother transferring bottles and syringes out of the plastic box. You might want to keep an extra set in the car or in a friend or relative's house.

Q. What would happen if you boiled the syringe or wiped it with spirit?

A. If you boiled a plastic syringe, it would disintegrate. If you wiped it with spirit you would rub off the numbers and after a few times it would fall apart. There is no need to sterilise it. If you replace the needle cover as soon as you have finished injecting, there is no way that bacteria will enter. It is quite safe.

Q. What about the glass syringe which is available on prescription?

A. The glass syringe may be boiled, of course, but it is usual to keep it in a plastic spirit case along with the needle.

Q. What kind of spirit is correct?

A. Industrial spirit.

Q. Is it necessary to boil the needles?

A. You may do so or you may keep them in spirit, but it is easier to use disposable needles and change them as often as necessary. Disposable needles are available on the Drug Tariff.

Q. Will my child always have to have injections?

A. If he is an insulin dependent diabetic, he will always have to have insulin. At the moment, the only insulin delivery system in general use is injection.

Q. Are two injections a day the most he will ever need?

A. Sometimes an extra injection is required during an illness to reduce a high blood sugar quickly. During pregnancy, better control can be acquired on three or even four injections. Most diabetics, however, need two injections a day, one before breakfast and one before the evening meal.

Q. Who should do the injections?

A. Ideally the diabetic himself should do them. If the child is very young, of course, the parent has to do them for him.

Q. At what age should a child do his own?

A. This varies with the ability and attitude of the child. I know children of six who do their own and are quite proud of their independence. I also know children many years older who refuse to look after their own diabetes or whose parents refuse to allow them to do it. I think that you should regard this in the same way that you regard other aspects of growing up. As soon as the child is able to take over, he should be allowed to do so. If you are looking for a simple answer, I think eight to ten years old is a reasonable age to expect this sort of independence.

Q. Should a child so young be allowed to fill the syringe?

A. Better to supervise this aspect of care for a few more years until you are certain that your child can do it without error. You will find that he will become quite expert in giving his injections in a short time. Again, I recommend most strongly that children be sent to a BDA holiday camp where these techniques can be perfected under medical supervision in a pleasant atmosphere.

3

Food Plan

Q. Why does my child have to be on a special diet?

A. In the non-diabetic, insulin production is automatic. Every time one eats, the correct amount of insulin is released. In the diabetic, this mechanism has failed. Insulin must be injected at least once a day. As the amount of insulin each day stays fairly consistent, so the amount of carbohydrate eaten should be approximately the same every day.

Q. What exactly is carbohydrate?

A. Food is designated as *carbohydrate*

protein

fat

Carbohydrate consists of sugars and starches. Examples of carbohydrate foods are cereals, bread, cake, biscuits, rice, pasta, barley, pulses like lentils, peas and beans, potatoes, fruit and milk products. Carbohydrate foods represent the bulk of our diet. They are generally the most filling and also the cheapest part of the food we eat.

Q. I thought that it was sugar which needed insulin. Bread and milk aren't sweet. Why do they need insulin?

A. All carbohydrates are broken down into simple sugars by the digestive system beginning with the saliva in the mouth and continuing with digestive juices in the small bowel. The main simple sugar carried in the blood is glucose and insulin is required for its use.

Q. Then why can't the diabetic avoid carbohydrate and eat only protein and fat to avoid the need for insulin?

A. Carbohydrate foods are necessary for good health and growth. A person who attempted to live on proteins and fats alone would not be well nourished. He would always be hungry. Bread, fruit and dairy products are an important part of our diet.

Q. Is a vegetarian diet suitable for diabetics?
A. Yes.

Q. Is it suitable for children?
A. It can be if sufficient protein is eaten. If your child is a vegetarian, the dietician in your clinic can help you to devise a vegetarian food plan suitable for your diabetic child.

Q. What sort of diet is suitable for diabetics?
A. Let's stop talking about 'diet', which has a negative connotation. Instead, let's call it a 'food plan'. A diabetic food plan is a good food plan for everyone in the family. In fact, this is really the secret of success in this aspect of diabetic control. Instead of restricting the diabetic child to a food plan which is suitable for him, change the eating habits of the family to conform to those recommended for the diabetic. You will find that the entire family will benefit.

Q. In what way?
A. There may be less obesity and risk of heart disease and possibly fewer bowel disorders.

Q. But doesn't my diabetic child have to be on a special diet?
A. He needs to be on a diet or food plan which *measures* the amount of carbohydrates taken rather than one which restricts it. Special diabetic diets which severely restict the amount of carbohydrate have gone out of fashion.

Modern diabetic food plans are suitable for everyone. The government, after a careful study of the relationship between illness and nutrition, have recommended that everyone reduce sugar, fat and salt and increase fibre. This applies both to diabetics and non-diabetics.

Q. How does this type of eating compare with our present diet?

A. Let's consider sugar. The average person in the UK consumes 5 ounces of sugar a day, about 10 tablespoons. Some of this is used for sweetening for coffee and tea but most of it is hidden in the processed food we buy.

Q. Do you mean cakes and puddings?

A. Yes, but also in breakfast cereals, tinned vegetables and meats, stock cubes, drinks, biscuits, crackers, bread, sauces, soups, gravy mixes, etc. Almost every food made in a factory contains sugar even if it does not taste sweet.

Q. Why is sugar put into foods which aren't meant to be sweet?

A. It is used as a preservative and to improve flavour.

Q. So, giving up sugar in coffee and tea isn't sufficient to reduce sugar intake, is it?

A. It will help, but it will not reduce it sufficiently to comply with recent government recommendations to reduce sugar consumption by a third unless we also reduce the amount of processed food we consume as well.

Q. What about fat? Why should fat reduction be important for diabetics?

A. For the same reason that it is important for non-diabetics, because there is strong evidence that there is less heart disease among populations whose fat consumption is lower than ours. Since diabetics are already at greater risk from heart disease of the arteries than non-diabetics, it seems sensible to reduce fat intake.

Q. What about salt?

A. Salt reduction is recommended where there is a risk of high blood pressure. Since diabetes can cause narrowing of the blood vessels which leads to high blood pressure in adult life, it is reasonable to reduce salt as well.

Q. I have heard a lot about fibre recently. What exactly is it and how is it important in diabetic eating plans?

A. Fibre is that part of plant foods which cannot be digested. It passes through the body and is eliminated. If it is removed, however, by modern refining methods for example, the food is assimilated more quickly and with less effort. The body doesn't have to work as hard. Muscles designed to deal with fibrous food become lax and very often problems ensue such as constipation, gall bladder trouble and bowel diseases.

Q. Are diabetics more likely to suffer from these diseases than non-diabetics?

A. Not necessarily, but these dietary changes are recommended for everyone. You are at a crossroads in your life at the moment where changes in diet are required. This would be a good time to introduce to your family better eating habits which will avoid these problems in the future. Also, since fibre rich foods take longer to be digested than those from which the fibre has been removed, they are a distinct advantage in controlling the blood glucose. The glucose levels in the blood rise more steeply after eating easily digested carbohydrate – like sweets and puddings than they do after eating foods such as wholemeal breads and cereals where the body has to work harder. You can use this natural phenomenon to help keep the blood glucose levels more even.

Q. What, then, is a good food plan for my child?

A. When a child is first diagnosed, it is usual for him to be admitted to hospital for stabilization. Often, his diabetes has caused him to lose weight, even become dehydrated and he is in need of specialized care for a few days. Insulin therapy will be started and he and his parents will have several consultations with the doctor and the dieticians. The dietician will discuss the family's eating patterns and recommend changes. Then the child will be given a food plan designed especially for him. This food plan will take into consideration his age, weight, preferences and dislikes, family circumstances and lifestyle. It will be worked out in conjunction with the amount and times of his insulin injections. The carbohydrates will be measured in grams and the amounts worked out for every meal.

Q. Is that very complicated?
A. Not at all. The dietician will tell you how many grams of carbohydrate are necessary for each meal and will help you to work out which foods would be most suitable. She will probably show you how to count exchanges.

Q. What are exchanges?
A. Exchanges are an easy way of adding up the carbohydrates. One exchange equals 10 grams of carbohydrate. An easy way to remember the amounts is to remember that each of the following equal one exchange:

  7 ounces of milk (average glass size)
  potato, the size of an egg
  1 packet potato crisps
  1 apple, pear, orange, small banana
  10 grapes
  1 plain yoghurt
  ½ fruit yoghurt
  small portion breakfast cereal (not sweetened)
  2 tbls rice
  2 tbls pasta (spaghetti, macaroni, lasagna, etc.)
  2 sausages
  6 dessertspoons of baked beans
  3 dessertspoons of spaghetti with sauce
  2 fish fingers
  1 small slice bread
  4 ounces unsweetened fruit juice

If, for example, four exchanges are recommended for breakfast, you might use any of these menus:

Breakfast Menu 1

bacon and egg	free – no exchanges
2 sausages	1 exchange
2 small slices toast with butter	2 exchanges
milk	1 exchange

Breakfast Menu 2

fresh orange	1 exchange
portion porridge	1 exchange
1 slice wholemeal bread and butter	1 exchange
milk	1 exchange

Breakfast Menu 3

4 ounces orange juice	1 exchange
portion corn flakes	1 exchange
2 small slices white bread toasted	1 exchange
tea without sugar	negligible carbohydrate

Breakfast Menu 4

high fibre cereal with banana slices	2 exchanges
1 slice wholemeal bread and butter	1 exchange
milk	1 exchange

All four of these menus contain 40 grams of carbohydrate or four exchanges each. Not all of them are equal in food value however. Menus 2 and 4 contain more high fibre, low fat foods. All these menus are suitable for a 4 exchange breakfast for your child, or anyone in the family but I should recommend that the foods in menus 2 and 4 be used more often than the foods in 1 and 3. There is no need to do this all at once. Gradual substitutions will hardly be noticed by the family and they can be weaned away from foods high in sugars, fats and salt gradually and quietly.

Q. *Does that mean that we shouldn't eat a cooked breakfast of bacon and eggs any more?*

A. Eat it if you enjoy it but don't eat it every day. Make it a special treat for Sundays and holidays. You will enjoy it all the more because it is a treat. And try serving the eggs scrambled, coddled or poached instead of fried. Grill the bacon and sausages instead of frying them. Use less butter or margarine.

Q. *What about jam? Should I get diabetic jam?*

A. If the amount of jam used is small (say, a teaspoonful), I wouldn't bother. If your child is very fond of jam and uses large quantities on his bread, you can get a sugarless variety. If your child likes jam sandwiches, try offering him a combination of peanut butter and jam. The peanut butter contains little sugar and the amount of jam used is much less than it would be on its own.

Q. What about other diabetic food?

A. I shouldn't bother with most of them. Generally, these are substitutions for very sweet foods which have little food value. It is better to work towards coaxing the family away from these foods into more healthy eating patterns than to reproduce the old habits using sugar substitutes. They can come in handy sometimes, however. If you are in the habit of distributing sweets to your children regularly, you can give a diabetic sweet to your diabetic child at these times. It is far better, though to give all your children fresh and dried fruits, nuts, low fat crisps and other sugarless treats instead of accustoming them to large amounts of sugar which causes tooth decay, poor appetite and may lead to other problems in the future.

Q. What about drinks?

A. Milk and fresh fruit juices have more food value than squashes whether sugarfree or full of sugar. Squashes are no more than sweetened coloured water and even the colouring agents may be harmful to some children who are sensitive to the chemicals used. If your children are used to drinking large amounts of squash, try making your own from fruit juice and water. The addition of ice and a slice of lemon can make these very attractive. For special treats, there are a number of sugarless drinks on the market either made or in a concentrated form to be mixed with water or made up in a soft drinks machine. Any diet drink can be used.

Q. What about puddings? My child loves puddings and would feel deprived without them. Are there special diabetic puddings available?

A. There are diabetic jellies on the market. These are similar to ordinary jellies except that they are made with artificial sweeteners instead of sugar. They are much more expensive however. I often make jelly from fruit juice and gelatine. This is quite delicious. You can drain the juice from a can of fruit (make sure that the fruit is tinned in juice not in syrup), prepare the jelly and when it is half set, add the fruit. A dollop of whipped cream on top makes it a pretty dessert for everyone. You can also use plain ice cream, fresh and dried fruit, small slice of plain cake, plain biscuits. With a bit of ingenuity almost any pudding can be made from ingredients which are lower in sugar. Half a peach or pear (tinned in fruit juice) in which is nestling a ball of plain ice cream topped with a small portion of whipped cream and a shaving of chocolate (diabetic chocolate is useful here) looks quite spectacular and should satisfy any child's yearning for a fancy pudding.

Q. *What about apple tart and custard, my family's favourite?*
A. If you bake the tart yourself, using wholemeal flour and fresh apples, you can improve the fibre content and decrease the sugar. You can mix the apple slices with fruit sugar (fructose – obtainable in health food shops or chemists) or artificial sweetener. You can make the custard yourself using fruit sugar again. This should reduce significantly the amount of sugar in the pudding. Puddings like this, however, should be served as treats for Sunday lunch and not as everyday fare. A piece of fresh fruit is a healthier dessert for everyday eating. If you save all the sweet foods for one day a week, you can increase the insulin dose slightly that day to cover it.

Q. *Is there a healthier substitute for custard? My family likes a jug of custard to pour over every slice of cake or pudding.*
A. Try fruit flavoured yoghurt as a topping for deserts. Try served baked apples with a spoonful of plain yoghurt on top. Don't make an issue of these things but try to increase the variety of their diet gradually by offering foods which look attractive.

Q. *Is yoghurt a permitted food for diabetics?*

A. Yes. There is at least one brand, too, which is low in fat and sugar. This is nice on its own or as a topping for fruit. Plain yoghurt with fresh bananas or berries is lovely. Strawberries and raspberries with yoghurt is just as nice as with cream and sugar. I think that you will find that once you begin to cut down on the sugar your taste buds will sharpen and other foods will taste better to you. After a time, you will detect the sugar hidden in processed foods which you never noticed before.

Q. *You mentioned fruit sugar. What is fruit sugar and how is it different from the sugar in the sugar packet?*

A. The sugar in the usual sugar packet is sucrose. It is made from sugar cane or beet, processed and refined. Fruit sugar or fructose is the natural sugar found in fruit. It also can be processed and refined. It is twice as sweet as sucrose so that only half the amount is required. It has been shown that diabetics can tolerate fructose better than sucrose. Small amounts of it do not cause the marked rise in blood glucose that is evident after eating sucrose. Still, doctors recommend that diabetics do not take more than 2 ounces a day. Use it sparingly in cooking. It is quite expensive compared with sucrose being about four times the price. I would recommend its use on special occasions only. For everyday cooking, try to eat fewer sugary foods.

The foods which are essential to good health are fresh fruit and vegetables, dairy products, cereal products (bread, rice, etc.) and meat, fish or poultry. (Vegetarians eat more vegetable protein to make up for eating no animal protein). None of these foods contains sugar. The sugar you buy in a packet is a completely unnecessary food. If you never bought another packet your health would never suffer from it. In fact, there is good evidence that it would improve. So consider all food made with sugar as extra to your basic food needs, pleasant for special treats but not essential to nutrition.

Q. *My child likes to sprinkle sugar on his morning cereal. Can fruit sugar be used?*

A. It is not recommended. Fruit sugar is useful in cooking but is too sweet for use on its own. Try slices of tinned or fresh fruit as a substitute. If all substitutes fail and your child is unhappy with his sugarless cereal, you can use Canderel Spoonful. This is an artificial sweetener made to look like sugar in a granulated form. I only recommend it (or any artificial sweetener) if all natural foods are rejected. You might offer a different breakfast until he stops yearning for sugared cereal. Dropped scones using wholemeal flour are a lovely breakfast and if you mix all the dry ingredients beforehand, you need only add milk, egg and butter to the mixture in the morning. It only takes a few minutes to mix the batter and drop it by the spoonful onto a greased griddle or frying pan. These pancakes can be served with diabetic jam. A plateful with a glass of milk and a fresh orange makes a nutritious breakfast or supper for any child.

If you have a waffle iron (some sandwich makers have waffle plates too), you can use the same batter to cook waffles. These waffles are far superior to the frozen waffles in the supermarket. The sugar suggested in the recipe books that accompany these waffle irons can be omitted. If you are really enterprising, you can bake stacks of waffles and freeze them. Then your child can reheat them in the toaster and be able to serve them to his friends just like the ready-made waffles. It is important that your child be able to entertain his friends in exactly the same way he would do if he were not diabetic. Making him different will always be detrimental to him.

Q. Can you recommend any other treats that my diabetic child can cook by himself?

A. He can make any American style ice cream soda by putting a spoonful of plain ice cream in a tall glass, adding sugar free soda and stirring until foamy. Serve with a straw and a long spoon. This is guaranteed to delight any young child and is a standby of mine for birthdays parties.

Q. What is the best thing to do for birthday parties? The food served is very sugary.

A. In my experience, the best thing to do is nothing. Let him enjoy himself. Birthday parties are rare occasions. The children expend so much energy running around playing that the excess carbohydrates will be used up. For the parties you give yourself, you can tailor the menu to suit your own ideas. For example, the cake does not have to be iced or frosted with sugar. You can use a plain cake and use ice cream on the top. Sugar-free drinks can be served or better yet, if you have a punch bowl, a pretty punch can be made from fresh juices, club soda, ice and fruit.

If you feel that you must distribute sweets, save them for going home. That way, the other children will be eating their chocolate bars on the way home and not in front of your youngster. Serve little bowls of nuts and crisps at the party instead of sweets. Children like grapes and mandarin oranges too. If, however, your child protests against any changes in the traditional party menu, don't worry. His birthday only comes once a year.

Q. *What about holidays with special foods like Christmas? Can my child eat Christmas cakes and chocolates?*

A. The BDA's magazine *Balance* always has recipes for Christmas cooking which are suitable for diabetics. Diabetic cookbooks have them as well. You can prepare these recipes or else give a thin sliver or the ordinary Christmas cake. If you allow these treats at the end of a meal rather than on their own as a between meal snack, they will not cause the blood glucose levels to rise as much. Also, you can increase the insulin dose on these occasions if you are concerned. Don't worry about this. With a bit of experience, you will know when to offer these foods and when to offer sugarless substitutes. There will be many times when your child's blood glucose will be low and when it will be in order for you to reach into the goody box for a special treat. The important thing to remember when your child is first diagnosed is that diabetes is for life. Hedging the child around with too many prohibitions will only make him rebellious and rebellion is the state that you want to avoid at all costs. Better to have the odd fluctuation in control than for him to turn against his condition at adolescence and refuse to look after himself.

Remember also that forbidden fruit is always sweeter. If you make a great show of hiding sweets and cakes to be eaten by the others when he is not around, you are only storing up problems for him in the future. If your child catches a glimpse of something he wants, give him a small piece and say nothing. If you think that it is extremely sugary, tell him that it is being saved for after dinner and give him a small piece then. Don't underline his condition by saying, as I have heard many mothers say, 'You can only have a little portion because you're a diabetic.' Give them all little portions and answer any complaints by telling them that too much sugar is bad for their teeth. After a while, you'll probably find that you will have fewer of these foods in the house. You will all get used to eating less sugar.

Q. My child's food plan given to us in hospital says that sweets and puddings are forbidden. Is this not so?

A. Your child's food plan is a guide for you both. It is not the gospel. Human beings are complex and far from perfect. Compromise is necessary in all human relations. There is a psychological element in all physical illness. An unhappy child is going to be more difficult to control. It is better to yield a little on these issues than to insist on perfection and push your child into rebelling against the diabetic regime.

Q. Can my child take school dinners or do I have to provide a packed lunch?

A. Either choice is appropriate. It is the carbohydrate content of the dinner which is important, not whether it comes from the school's kitchen or from yours. If your child enjoys taking school dinners, I should let him continue. There is usually more involved than the actual eating of the meal. Often the choice of whether to take dinners or bring them has social ramifications. The children divide themselves up at meal time, sit with certain friends, spend a certain amount of time in the playground or doing their homework. These patterns establish themselves early in the school term. Changing from one option to another in the middle of the term may be upsetting. If he is used to taking school dinners, it would be better to check that the carbohydrate content is suitable, make any changes necessary and then let him go on as usual.

Q. How can I determine the carbohydrate content?

A. Get a list of the school menus from the Head Master. If you cannot estimate the carbohydrate on offer yourself, the clinic dietician will be able to help you. You will probably find that it is more than sufficient for your child's midday needs. Undoubtedly the pudding is too sweet but the rest of the dinner will fit in to his regime. In that case, if your child can be trusted to substitute fresh fruit or a yoghurt for the pudding, give him some to keep in his schoolbag. If you think that the temptation to eat the pudding will be more than he can resist, you can speak to the school authorities about substituting a more suitable dessert for him or else changing to a packed lunch. You should, however, discuss the matter with your child. If he is old enough to stay in school during the lunch hour, he is old enough to have a preference. Be tactful. Try to arrive at a mutually agreed solution. This will avoid the situation where the child eats the school pudding surreptitiously, setting a pattern for future deception and promoting the eating of unsuitable food to an act of defiance against his parents.

Also, it is important to prevent the school, in a misguided attempt to be helpful, to embarrass your child by making an issue of the fact that he has to eat special food. He doesn't and they shouldn't be allowed to think that he does. I have heard tales of the over zealous 'dinner lady' who would snatch away a dish of ice cream from under the nose of a diabetic child crying, 'You can't have that, you're diabetic' or the one who herded several diabetic children together at a separate table shouting at them as they entered the dining hall, 'Diabetics this way'. This kind of well meaning but tactless behaviour on the part of the school staff can hurt your child's feelings. Diabetes will be a blow to him. Having to inject himself will be a trauma. You don't want to add an additional trauma by making him feel different or an invalid.

Q. If I give my child a packed lunch, what should I pack?
A. First, you must look at the food plan that he has received from the dietician or the doctor. How many exchanges does it recommend? (In some clinics, exchanges are called lines or portions. The basic unit, though, is ten grams of carbo-hydrate. The name is unimportant). If it recommends 4 exchanges (40 grams) of carbohydrate, you might choose from among menus like these:

Packed lunch 1

sandwich made with two pieces of white bread from small loaf filled with chopped egg, tinned fish, cheese, peanut butter, sliced meat, etc.	2 exchanges
a piece of fruit	1 exchange
tin of sugarless soda	free
2 plain biscuits	1 exchange

Packed lunch 2

sandwich made with two slices wholemeal bread filled with chopped egg, tinned fish, cheese, peanut butter, sliced meat, etc.	2 exchanges
fruit	1 exchange
fruit juice in carton	1 exchange

Packed lunch 3

Thermos of soup (creamed or fairly thick with vegetables, lentils, barley, etc.)	1 exchange
wholemeal scone or bun with butter	1 exchange
cheese	free

FOOD PLAN

fruit	1 exchange
sugarless drink	free
low fat crisps	1 exchange

Packed lunch 4

Thermos of stew with meat, vegetables and potatoes	1–2 exchanges depending on amount of potato (see page 37.)
salad of fresh vegetables	free
fruit	1 exchange
fruit juice	1 exchange
2 plain biscuits if necessary	

You can see that these menus all have the same carbohydrate value but menus 3 and 4 include a hot dish and menu 2 is preferable to menu 1 because of the choice of bread.

Q. What about break time?

A. It is fortunate that all schools allow time for between-meal snacks so that the diabetic's need for frequent meals is shared by all the children. Most primary schools provide milk at break time. Milk and two plain biscuits is generally sufficient. You can vary the menu by sending a banana instead of the biscuits or a packet of crisps. Whatever you choose, try to make it the same as the things the other children take.

Q. Suppose that the other children take sweets?

A. If the others take sweets, give your child a packet of diabetic sweets but include a piece of fruit or a bag of crisps so that he will have enough carbohydrate. I think that you will find that most of the children bring biscuits to have with their milk and not sweets. Your child's teacher will be able to advise you.

Q. Does he need an afternoon snack too?

A. Yes. He needs to eat something every two and a half to three hours. Most children, however, diabetic and non-diabetic, do this. If he lives near the school and comes straight home, he can have his afternoon snack at home. If he has to travel home by bus or if he stays in school to play or for any after school activity, he should have his break with him in his schoolbag.

Q. What sort of food is best?

A. If he requires 2 exchanges at this time (again, consult your food plan) any of the following are in order: plain yoghurt and fruit, sandwich, milk and two plain biscuits, cereal and fruit, low fat crisps and an apple, plain cake with tea, bread and butter, etc. Most foods are appropriate. Don't give him ice lollies or other sugary treats at this time, however. Eaten on a comparatively empty stomach, they tend to send the blood glucose up. Starchy foods which take longer to be digested are better for afternoon snacks. Save the ice lolly for the occasional after-meal treat.

Q. What sort of food is suitable for the evening meal?

A. This depends on whether or not the midday meal or his dinner is the main meal of the day. If the evening meal is dinner for all the family, the usual combination of meat, vegetables and potatoes (or rice or pasta) with fruit or a simple pudding is as suitable for him as for the other children in the family. This meal is entirely under your control so you can make the most of it as a way of introducing healthier eating habits for everyone. Try serving fish or poultry more often than meat and increase fresh vegetables, lightly cooked or raw. Small children usually love raw carrot sticks and celery stalks. Encourage this. If your family insists on chips, drain them well with kitchen roll or clean brown paper bags. Cut them thick. The thin ones absorb more oil. Don't use the oil more than twice. With each lot you fry, the oil becomes more saturated. Try to serve steamed or boiled potatoes instead for some of the meals. If your child's carbohydrate allowance for the evening meal is 6 exchanges, any of the following menus contain that amount. In measuring the amount of carbohydrate in potatoes, remember that a potato the size of an egg contains 10 grams or 1 exchange.

FOOD PLAN

Menu 1

clear soup	free
meat, fish or poultry	free
baked potato (6 ounces)	3 exchanges
boiled carrots	free
milk	1 exchange
ice cream and tinned peach half	2 exchanges

Menu 2

vegetable soup or other thick soup	1 exchange
omelette	free
chips (6 ounces)	3 exchanges
small portion baked beans	1 exchange
milk	1 exchange
sugarless jelly	free

Menu 3

fresh vegetable salad	free
spaghetti or other pasta	
6 rounded tbls	3 exchanges
slice garlic bread	1 exchange
plain ice cream	1 exchange
milk	1 exchange

Menu 4

beefburger	free
chips (6 ounces)	3 exchanges
tea	free
2 small slices toast	2 exchanges
piece of fruit	1 exchange

Menu 5

curry with rice (2 tbls = 10 grams)	4 exchanges
lentil dahl (small portion)	1 exchange
1 chapatti	1 exchange
sugarless drink or tea	free

Menu 6

2 slices bacon (grilled)	free
2 sausages	1 exchange

mushrooms and tomatoes	free
egg	free
3 small slices bread with butter	3 exchanges
tea	free
plain cake or 2 biscuits	2 exchanges

Q. Can you suggest a list of foods which I can safely give my child and tell me how much carbohydrate they contain?

A. Here is a partial list. (The BDA have a large list called *Countdown* which tells you the carbohydrate values of manufactured foods. It also suggests which of these foods can be eaten freely and which should be eaten less frequently. It can be bought from them.)

Foods with no carbohydrate
meat, poultry, fish (without breading)
eggs
green vegetables
sugar-free drinks
hard cheese (like cheddar)
mayonnaise
spices

Food with very little carbohydrate (less than 10 grams per serving)
carrots
peas (fresh or frozen but not dried)
frozen fish in sauce
frankfurters
beefburgers
prawn cocktail

Food with 10 grams of carbohydrate (1 exchange)
1 small slice bread
potato, the size of an egg
7 thick chip shop chips
spaghetti, macaroni, lasagne, etc. 2 rounded tbls
rice (boiled or steamed) 2 tbls
porridge oats (½ ounce uncooked)

breakfast cereals (unsweetened) ½ ounce
yoghurt (natural) 1 pot
yoghurt (fruit flavoured) ½ pot
2 fish fingers
2 sausages
1 fish cake
fried fish in breading (1 ounce)
¼ frozen fish pie
2 ounces sweet corn
4 tbls baked beans
5 ounces broad beans
5 tbls kidney beans
½ Jordan's Original Crunchy Bar
⅓ can apple slices in juice
2 rings pineapple in juice
2 pear halves in juice
2 peach halves in juice
1 frozen waffle
2 ginger thins
1 digestive biscuit
2 Marie biscuits
4 Ritz crackers
5 cheddar crackers
3 Tuc crackers
2 cream crackers
2 thin arrowroot biscuits
2 Nice biscuits
1 bag potato crisps

Q. What foods have to be eliminated completely?
A. No foods. All foods have their place, even sweets. The sensible way to handle requests for foods you feel are inappropriate is to suggest that they be saved for another time. If your child's diabetes is being carefully controlled, there will be many times when his blood glucose will be low and a sweet will be the best way to bring it up to normal. He should always carry something sweet in his pocket for these occasions.

Q. How can I be certain that the sweet in his pocket won't find its way into his mouth at the wrong time?

A. The only way that you can be reasonably certain of this is by discussing it with your child. Unless he is very small, he can be taught about food values. His desire to cheat is usually fuelled by his normal and natural need to assert his independence. If you allow him as much independence as is appropriate for a child of his age, he will be less likely to sneak inappropriate foods in order to feel grown up. It is also a good idea to stop buying these foods. It is grossly unfair to forbid a child to help himself to sugary biscuits when the kitchen cupboard is overflowing with them. If you enjoy cooking, try baking these things at home. You can use healthier ingredients and less sugar if you do. If cooking is not your scene or if the time in the kitchen is limited, perhaps there is someone else in the family who enjoys cooking and would be pleased to bake for you. Often, a grandmother or other relative or friend would be only too delighted to feel useful in this way. In addition to the obvious benefits of having a supply of home baked foods, there is also a great psychological boost from sharing this problem. Looking after a diabetic child is very taxing emotionally. There is no respite from worry. There is much benefit to be gained from involving another adult in this concern.

Q. Somebody told me that her dietician forbids all canned soups. I do not have the time to cook soup. What can I do?

A. The first thing you can do is to stop listening to everyone's advice. If you don't, you will end up hedged around with hundreds of prohibitions, most of them based on half truths and misconceptions. There are many different types of canned soups. Some are clear soups, bouillons and con-sommés which have very little food value but which might have quite a bit of added sugar. If the second ingredient on the label is sugar you can be reasonably certain that the sugar content is high and the food value low. You would probably not be giving these to your children anyway. Soups with vegetables and meat have varying carbohydrate values. Here is a list of some which contain approximately 10 grams of carbohydrate (1 exchange) and can be used fairly freely.

Packet soups which make 1 pint
(a portion here would be ⅓ pint)

vegetable and beef	minestrone
barbecue beef and tomato	oxtail
chicken and mushroom	scotch broth
chicken noodle	
thick chicken	
golden vegetable	

Instant soups (like Cup-a-Soup) (a portion is the entire packet)

chicken noodle	most low calorie soups
onion and beef	

Canned soups (½ can = 1 portion)

cream of vegetable	mushroom
oxtail	chicken

Condensed soups (⅓ can = 1 portion)

chicken noodle	cream of mushroom
cream of celery	cream of tomato
cream of chicken	stock pot

These soups can be used but, naturally, the soups you make at home will be less expensive, probably tastier, free from additives like colouring agents and taste boosters, and you will control the amount of carbohydrate. I think that your friend's dietician was urging her to use less convenience food. This is certainly a good idea. It really takes very little time to cook a large pot of soup once or twice a week. It is an economic way of using leftovers too. It is also a good way to ensure that your family gets plenty of fresh vegetables – especially if yours is a family which doesn't like vegetables other than frozen peas or baked beans.

Q. *Are all convenience foods to be omitted?*
A. It is hard to make general rules which apply to everyone.

Convenience foods have multiplied lately due, in part, to the fact that fewer women are full-time homemakers now. Avoiding all convenience foods would be extremely difficult for most people. But it is also true that many people who do have time to cook and enjoy cooking have fallen into the habit of using convenience foods just because they are there, arrayed temptingly on the supermarket shelves or in the freezers. Next time you go to the supermarket take a critical look at your shopping basket before you reach the checkout desk. Do you really need to buy that frozen pie? What happened to the delicious pies you used to make? Are all those tinned and frozen vegetables good value? Fresh vegetables in season are tastier and have a nicer texture. Read labels carefully. You will be amazed to learn how many convenience foods are full of water and chemicals.

You may be spending your money on things that aren't even foods. Not only are you giving your diabetic child foods in which there is a substantial amount of hidden sugar but you are giving all the family foods which contain chemical substances which are unknown to most of us. Some are even forbidden in other countries. Additives marked with E are allowed in Europe. Those without E are not. Some of the food which we are buying is not allowed to be sold in other countries in the EEC. Why? To answer your question simply, use convenience foods if you have to but try to incorporate more fresh foods and home made dishes into your family's eating plan. That way, you will know more precisely what you are serving them.

Q. Does my child need a bedtime snack?
A. Yes. It is normal for the blood glucose levels to fall during the night. A good idea for bedtime snacks is to take something which will not be too quickly absorbed by the body. Milk with wholemeal bread or cereal is a good choice.

Q. What about cocoa?
A. Milky drinks are fine but choose a brand of cocoa without added sugar. Artificial sweeteners can be used. There are

some brands of milky drinks which are reduced in calories for dieters. Try one of these.

Q. *What do you think about diabetic chocolate Easter eggs or Santas?*

A. These products are sweetened with sorbitol. Large amounts of sorbitol can cause diarrhoea. If small bits are eaten at a time, there is no harm in them. If, however, your child will eat the entire confection at one sitting, he will get more sorbitol than is wise. One Christmas product which is more manageable than a chocolate Santa Claus is a little sack of diabetic chocolate coins wrapped in gold paper. You can put a few of these in his Christmas stocking and give one or two a day over the holiday period when the other children are being given gifts of chocolate.

Q. *What about other types of diabetic chocolate? Are they all sweetened with sorbitol?*

A. There are one or two brands of chocolate which are made with fructose. These are quite nice. They taste much more like ordinary chocolate. They are useful for grating over desserts too. Generally, however, I should regard these sweets as special treats and not offer them often. Try to wean the family away from the idea that a treat means a sweet. It is better to spend your money on healthier foods. A watermelon in the summer can be offered as a special treat. And it is one which can be eaten by all the family. Similarly, cherries, fresh apricots, kiwi fruits, strawberries, melons, etc. can be regarded as special foods for special occasions.

Q. *What about alcohol? I like to cook in wine sometimes.*

A. When you heat wine, the alcohol virtually disappears. Only the taste remains. Besides, the amount in one portion is negligible. This method of cooking is perfectly all right from the point of view of carbohydrate content.

Q. *Besides exotic fruits, what other foods are useful for treats?*

A. Popcorn is one of my favourites. You should not add sugar, however. Freshly popped corn with a bit of melted butter on the top is popular with my child and her friends. Nuts, Twiglets, corn and potato crisps (low fat if available), plain ice cream (sprinkle grated diabetic chocolate over it to make it special), waffles topped with ice cream or sugarless maple syrup, cheese straws made with wholemeal flour, homemade biscuits made with wholemeal flour and reduced in sugar, diet drinks. You can jazz things up to make them appealing to a child by many simple methods.

It is my experience that anything served with a straw is more enjoyable to a child than the same drink without a straw. A slice of fruit on top of a simple dessert makes it fancy. Ice cubes have great charisma. Ice cubes with something frozen in the middle like a sprig of mint or a tiny cherry decorate a glass of simple fruit punch and make it a special treat. Be inventive. There is no end to this sort of creativity. If you think about it in a positive way, your child need not feel deprived of the normal pleasures of childhood eating.

Q. *Can you tell me what kind of foods which have low sugar or low fat are stocked in an ordinary supermarket?*

A. More of these foods are stocked today than were a year or two ago because of the greater interest today in healthier eating. There are also television programmes which discuss this issue and offer many worthwhile suggestions. Some of these shows produce fact sheets which can be obtained. Some have cookbooks which you can buy. Here is a list of the low fat and low sugar foods which are available in my local supermarket.

Low fat
 various spreads made from buttermilk, or a combination of milk and oil

low fat cheeses	low fat salad dressings
reduced fat sausages	diet cocoa
low fat potato crisps	skim milk
low fat mayonnaise	frozen diet dinners

Low Sugar

diet drinks	reduced sugar bacon
fruits tinned in juice or water	diet soups

Besides these foods, however, you have the entire range of fresh fruits and vegetables, wholemeal breads and cereals, lean meats, fish, poultry, cottage cheese, etc. that are naturally low in sugar and fat and high in food value.

4

Diabetes in the Very Young

Q. How can diabetic control be measured in the very young child?

A. Urine can be tested by squeezing out a wet nappie on to a testing strip. Disposable nappies are best for this purpose as there is no danger of soap or detergent affecting the chemistry of the urine. Blood tests can also be done. Most babies and young children submit to blood tests with fairly good grace. Make sure that the little fingers are warm so that the blood comes easily.

Q. Is caring for him very difficult?

A. Because diabetes is quite unusual in very young children, often the diagnosis isn't made until the child has become quite ill, usually dehydrated. He will be put on a drip in hospital. After discharge, he still may be thin and debilitated. Often his appetite is poor. He may be cranky. Injections and blood tests will irk him further. Looking after him will be difficult until he has recovered health and spirits. Parents will worry about whether or not he is eating enough. The diet sheet provided by the hospital is a good guide. Frequent testing is another. If the family can possibly afford household help, this is the time to get it, even if it is just a teenage girl to come in after school and play with the child or children or talk them for a walk. Caring for a young diabetic is exhausting.

Q. How can such a child be coaxed to eat all the carbohydrate that he needs if his appetite is poor?

A. Small meals offered frequently go down better than larger ones at longer intervals. Give a snack before nap time. Make the food look as attractive as possible to tempt him. Finger food might be more appealing to a little child than a formal presentation on a plate. Bananas, plain biscuits, low sugar rusks, milk blended with egg, orange and sugar are useful standbys. If you have an electric blender, you can blend a banana with milk and ice cream to get a tempting drink which is rich in carbohydrates. It may be that his insulin has to be reduced as his health improves and he becomes more active.

Q. *If the child is too young to recognise the warning signals of a hypo, how can they be avoided?* (Hypoglycaemia or 'hypo' is low blood glucose. For a discussion of the symptoms and what to do, see p 80 and Appendix 2 on p 110.)

A. The parent has to be extra observant. If his nap is longer than usual, be suspicious. (Always give food before a nap.) If he loses colour or becomes listless after playing happily for a time, check his blood sugar. If possible, make sure that someone is watching him all the time. The other family members can take this in turn. If there are older children, they might be able to do this.

Q. *Is it best to keep him close to home?*

A. Not necessarily. Children who are carted around to suit their parents' convenience usually turn out to be more easy going and flexible than those who are guarded at home. Whatever you do, however, whether it is staying at home or going out, carry food with you. No diabetic should venture out of doors without some sugar available to him. Carry sugar, biscuits and fruit in your handbag at all times. A simple way of carrying sugar is to buy Dextrasol tablets. These are squares of glucose which are quickly absorbed by the body. They are made in various fruit flavours and are available in most chemists. Athletes use them often for quick energy. An older child can carry his own. They come in a neat packet which is easily carried in a pocket. Packets can be left in the car to deal with any threatened hypos.

5

At School

Q. Shall I tell my child's teacher that he is a diabetic?

A. You should tell the teacher and the Head as well. They must know what to do if your child's blood glucose gets too low at school. The BDA produce a leaflet called 'The Diabetic at School'. It costs 10p. They also have a School Pack which gives much information in an accessible form. This literature will help to answer questions about your child's food plan, his need for between meal snacks and whether or not he can play games.

Another person who needs to know that your child has developed diabetes is the bus driver. If he should become ill on the school bus, the driver needs to know what to do. Give the bus driver a sweet drink like fruit juice or lucozade to keep handy for emergencies. Give him a packet of biscuits as well. If the bus breaks down and has to wait for repairs, the driver should be aware that this delay might cause a problem for the diabetic child. He should know enough about diabetes to make certain that the child is all right and to advise him to eat a snack. Your child, of course, should always have food in his schoolbag for unforeseen events.

Q. Is it safe for my child to participate in strenuous games?

A. There is no reason for the diabetic to refrain from playing any sort of game. On the contrary, exercise is an important part of the control of diabetes. A few precautions are necessary, however. He should take extra carbohydrate before strenuous exercise and more afterward. If he is swimming hard, a mini Mars bar before entering the pool and an apple or a sandwich when he gets out will keep his blood glucose from dropping below normal. (Just fooling around in the pool is not hard work. Extra carbohydrate is only needed for sustained effort.)

Q. What about competitive sport? Suppose he wants to be a member of the school team which competes against other schools. This can be extremely strenuous and may take place away from home.

A. Your child must learn to live with his diabetes. If his athletic ability is such that he is chosen to represent his school, this is an important achievement for him. It would be wrong and foolish to forbid him to take the place that he has earned. He would feel a failure and an invalid. That is exactly what you want to avoid. Let him go, of course, but make sure that a few basic rules are followed.

> 1 *He must take enough food to cover all meals and snacks at their usual hours.* (This is something that all the children will be doing anyway. The bus resounds with the crunch of crisps on these occasions.)
> 2 *He must take extra carbohydrate for the match both before and after.*
> 3 *He must tell someone about his diabetes.* This person could be his friend.

The friend can be invaluable to the diabetic child. When the blood sugar drops below normal, the diabetic usually becomes fractious. He may not be aware that he needs food. He has to be reminded. The friend sitting next to him is the ideal person to do this. I have heard my child's friend say many a time, 'You'd better eat something. You're horribly cross.' The teacher or group leader should be told about his diabetes too but he will be glad to rely on the observations of the friend. With a bit of help from these two, your child can take his place on the team. There are quite a few athletes, even Olympic competitors, who are diabetic.

Q. Should I give my child's teacher Lucozade or a similar drink to keep in the classroom?

A. Yes, that's a good idea. The sugar in Lucozade, Coca Cola, orange or pineapple juice is rapidly absorbed. There are many individual-sized drinks on the market today. These are packed with a straw attached to the carton which makes them very handy. They are useful for the teacher's desk and also for the child's bedside table. (If he feels 'hypo' in the night he can drink it.) A quick-thinking teacher can head off a situation which could be embarrassing for the child. It is difficult for a child to have to return to class the day after he has been making a spectacle of himself, perhaps causing the other children to laugh at him. Such a situation only reinforces the idea that he is different, that he cannot function away from Mummy and Daddy, that life is dangerous away from home.

Q. *Why is exercise so important?*

A. It requires large amounts of glucose for fuel. If this glucose were not required by activity, it would accumulate in the blood stream where it would cause trouble. Exercise keeps the blood glucose levels lower. A diabetic who takes regular exercise will find it invaluable in keeping glucose levels normal or close to normal. Children enjoy vigorous activity and the diabetic child should be encouraged to partake every day.

Q. *In the winter, it is almost dark when my child returns from school. With homework and television, there is little time for sport. How can this situation be changed?*

A. Perhaps cycling to and from school is the answer. Perhaps he can walk further to get the school bus or he can be dropped from the car further from the school building. If none of these ideas is suitable, how about introducing some sort of family exercise session at home? There are many tapes and videos of aerobics, yoga and other sort of exercising. Don't treat this as part of his diabetic therapy. Introduce it as fun for the family and healthy for father's middle-aged spread or mother's desire to fit into her bikini.

Q. *Is there any type of exercise which is not suitable for diabetics?*

A. Scuba diving, parachuting and motor racing are best left alone. In fact, the British Sub Aqua Club and the British

Parachute Association discourage insulin-dependent diabetics. In these sports, a hypo might be fatal. Swimming alone is dangerous for anyone but especially for diabetics. He should always have a companion and have easy access to sugar should he feel his sugar levels falling. But with proper precautions, swimming is excellent exercise and should not be discouraged.

Q. *How could one have easy access to sugar while swimming?*
A. Perhaps a small leak-proof plastic box could house a few glucose tablets or sweets. This could be left at the side of the pool or even tucked into the swimming costume. Eating a small bar of chocolate before a long swim is easy enough to do and generally will suffice.

Q. *Are there any special problems about school?*
A. One aspect of diabetic care which the school must know about is the necessity for meals to be eaten on time. Generally, this is easily managed in schools as it is important for the school timetable to adhere to a strict schedule. Occasionally, there can be a problem which is better avoided than coped with after it happens. The teacher must understand that deprivation of food cannot be tolerated by the diabetic. He cannot miss his snack or his lunch. Depriving him of food can never be used as a method of punishment. He must be allowed to dip into his school bag for snacks even if this is not generally allowed in class. Accordingly, he must be allowed to take food into the examination room if he is taking a lengthy examination. If the school has more than one period for lunch, he must be consulted as to which meal time will suit him best. If his lunch must be a late one because of schedule conflicts, he must be allowed to eat something extra in his classroom.

Q. *Should a school-age diabetic wear an ID bracelet?*
A. This question is a difficult one. Ideally, yes. All diabetics, especially an older child travelling to school on a public bus or walking or cycling a long distance, are better protected with

an ID bracelet or necklace. In practice, however, it doesn't always work out that way. After my child 'lost' three ID necklaces and a half dozen cards, I finally realised that she resented wearing or carrying one. Children can be extremely sensitive about anything which sets them apart from the others.

I think that your child ought to be consulted in this matter if he is old enough to have an opinion about it. It may be that a young child will be indifferent to the issue or will like wearing it. Some older children might like wearing one too. If the child is resistant, however, I wouldn't persist in this. If you encounter resistance to the idea of a necklace or bracelet, perhaps an ID card in the pocket of the school uniform and all sports clothes would be acceptable.

Q. Where are identifying cards and jewellery obtained?

A. Your diabetic clinic probably has ID cards. They are usually given away by the companies which make diabetic supplies. Your local BDA branch may have them too. If you can't get hold of one, try the nearest Boots, the Chemists. I believe that they have a stock of them. The ID jewellery is advertised in *Balance*. I believe that Boots have a range of them as well. You can write to a company called Medic-Alert which supplies the jewellery and also keeps your child's medical requirements on file. In case of accident, a doctor or nurse can contact them (number on the disc) and find out what your child's normal insulin dosage is. Of course you must keep them informed of any changes.

Q. I have heard that stress should be avoided by diabetics. Should my child be discouraged from attempting difficult exams at school so as to reduce the stress on him?

A. Your child is diabetic, true, but he is also a person, potential worker, parent and spouse. Education is as important to him as to the non-diabetic. Diabetes should not be an inhibiting factor in his academic achievement. A recent study of school children has shown no difference in levels of achievement between the diabetic and the non-diabetic child. Your child should not be encouraged to use his diabetes as an excuse for poor school performance.

In fact, if he realises (and many children are very quick to realise their advantages) that he can manipulate the teacher with his diabetes by using it as an excuse for homework not completed, exams missed, etc., he will turn his attention to you as well. Parents can be manipulated by children very easily. This situation is bad for everyone but the results are especially destructive for the child. He is not an invalid (if you don't make him one) and can cope with school stresses as well as the non-diabetic child.

Q. Is boarding school advisable for the diabetic child?

A. If the reasons for which the child is boarding are those unconnected with his diabetes, I think that the problem of boarding can be overcome with a bit of forethought. In the boarding situation, the staff have to be fully aware of any possible problems. Whoever will be in charge of the dormitory or bedrooms at night must know that a night-time hypo is possible and know what to do about it. The child must be allowed to keep food and drink at his bedside at night even if this is usually against the school rules. The school must be prepared for the occasional unpleasant, even frightening incident of a night-time hypo and understand that the unreasonable behaviour which accompanies these episodes is not to be held against the child. Also, the school food must be examined carefully. Is it suitable for the diabetic child? Very often, school food is disliked. The child may eat less than he needs and a hypo may follow. The child who is boarding must be responsible enough to understand that he has to finish his dinner even if he dislikes the food or else must ask for and receive a substitute.

It is unreasonable for anyone to expect that the school cook will prepare a different meal to suit one child but perhaps it can be arranged that bread and butter and a glass of milk will be forthcoming in that situation. If it is usual that all the children in the family attend boarding schools then I think that the effort should be made to control the diabetes in the boarding situation.

It is very important that diabetes should not be seen as a factor which will change everyone's life. It is disruptive enough without making everything else in the family's life subordinate to it. No one benefits from that sort of attention least of all the diabetic child. On the other hand, if boarding school is being considered for the child *because* he is diabetic, in other words because parents fear that they cannot cope with the situation, I think that the remedy is too drastic. The child will resent being sent away because he has presented his parents with a problem which they cannot solve. He has a right to expect that his parents will be able to cope with his diabetes at home.

Q. Now that my child has become diabetic, should he be allowed to participate in very strenuous games at school like football?

A. Exercise is an important part of good diabetic control. The best exercise for anyone is the one that he enjoys most. If football is a favourite activity he should be allowed to play football. Since it is so strenuous, it will be necessary to take a few simple precautions so that his blood glucose does not drop below normal. A snack before the match and a snack afterwards is generally all that is needed. Diabetes is not a bar to athletic achievement. Diabetics have participated in sport up to Olympic levels.

Q. What about activities like Outward Bound, which are not only strenuous but may involve danger and require self-reliance?

A. Find out more about these activities. If your child will be accompanied by another person and if food and drink can be carried, it is probably all right. If your child likes this kind of activity, the BDA have an Outward Bound type of camp for teenagers in Scotland. Water sports is the speciality there. You can find out more about it by writing to the Youth Department. I do not think that activities which require a solo effort in remote places are suitable for diabetics. He really needs to be accompanied by another person in case his blood glucose drops below normal. In that situation, perhaps also cold and wet, his mental capacities will be affected temporarily and he may not be able to take the necessary steps to bring his glucose levels up to normal. He needs a companion who will recognise the signs of hypoglycaemia and insist that he eat or drink something.

6

Control

Q. Throughout, you have emphasised good control, but how can this control be measured?

A. It can be measured by testing the urine and/or the blood to determine how much glucose is present. It can also be measured by testing the urine for the presence of ketones.

Q. Can these tests be peformed at home?
A. Yes.

Q. Is special equipment necessary?
A. Yes, but it is easily obtained. Equipment for testing urine for glucose or ketones is available on prescription. There are two methods of doing this at the moment – reagent strips and tablets.

1 Testing by reagent strips

This is the simplest method. Get a bottle of reagent strips from the chemist. The most common brand is Diastix.

Wet the end of the strip with urine by passing it through the urine stream for 2 seconds. Boys can do this easily, of course. Girls can do it too with a bit of care. If girls find it difficult, however, they can catch the urine in a little basin or jar and dip the strip into it.

Wait 30 seconds exactly. Shake the excess urine off the strip. Immediately compare the coloured patch on the end of the strip with the colour chart on the bottle. The coloured square that best matches the test area tells you how much glucose is present in the urine.

2 Testing for glucose with reagent tablets

(A) 5 Drop Method

Get a bottle of reagent tablets from the chemist. The most

common brand is called Clinitest. It consists of a bottle of tablets, a test tube and a plastic dropper.

Catch the urine in a jar or basin. Fill the dropper and put 5 drops of the urine into the test tube.

Discard the rest of the urine and wash the dropper.

Add 10 drops of water to the test tube.

Put one Clinitest tablet into the test tube. Do not touch it with your fingers. The easiest way to handle the tablets is to shake one into the bottle cap and gently tip it into the tube. Recap the bottle immediately.

Holding the test tube at the top (it will get hot) watch the liquid foam up and change colour.

Fifteen seconds after boiling has stopped, shake the tube gently and immediately compare the colour with the chart on the Clinitest packet.

(B) 2 Drop Method

This method is sometimes recommended to test higher levels of glucose. If your doctor recommends the 2 Drop Method, you proceed in the same way using only 2 drops of urine and 10 drops of water. A special colour chart for use with this method is inside the packet. It is available on prescription.

3 Testing for ketones by reagent strips

Get a bottle of strips from the chemist. The commonest brand is called Ketostix. It is available on prescription. Wet the strip in the same way. Wait thirty seconds. 'Read' the strip by comparing it to the colour chart on the bottle.

4 Testing for ketones with reagent tablets

Get a bottle of Acetet tablets available on prescription from the chemist.

Collect urine in a jar or basin.

Shake one tablet out onto the washhandbasin. Do not touch it with your fingers.

With the dropper, place one drop of urine on the tablet. Compare the colour change with the chart in the packet.

Q. What are ketones and why do you have to test for them?
A. Ketones are fatty acids in the body. If the body is unable to use glucose (because of lack of insulin), it breaks down fat molecules and ketones are released. If the urine shows evidence of ketones, it is a sign that more insulin is required.

Q. What is acetone? In the hospital, they tested for acetones. Is this the same as ketones?
A. Acetone is one type of ketone.

Q. How often should you test the urine?
A. Unless you are directed differently by your doctor, I should test once a day for glucose and if all is well, once a week for ketones. If glucose is found in the urine though, it would be a good idea to test it for ketones as well. During illness, it is important to test the urine more frequently.

Q. What is a normal reading?
A. A normal reading shows no glucose or ketones in the urine. It is not an entirely accurate guide, however, because glucose normally does not spill over into the urine until the levels in the blood are quite a bit higher than normal. The absence of glucose in the urine test really means that the level of glucose in the blood is below 10 mmol/l, the level at which it first appears in the urine. The normal range in the blood, however, is between 4 mmol/l and 7 mmol/l approximately. A negative reading in the urine test, then, only tells us that the blood glucose is less than 10 mmol/l. It cannot tell us whether the blood glucose is slightly elevated, say between 8 and 10 mml/l or whether it is below normal (below 4 mml/l) and the child is in danger of having a hypoglycaemic reaction. Urine testing is useful, especially in illness, but it is a tool with limited use.

Q. Are there other methods of testing?
A. Yes, blood testing gives more information

Q. Can blood be tested at home?

A. Yes. The single most important advance in the control of diabetes since the discovery of insulin in 1921 is the measurement of blood glucose at home. The technique is simple and with it the diabetic can alter his insulin and diet to achieve glucose levels which are near normal most of the time.

Q. What equipment is required?
A. All that is required is a needle or automatic pricker to obtain the drop of blood, blood testing reagent strips (similar to those used for urine testing) and a watch with a second hand. A reflectance meter or machine to read the strips by is optional. The procedure is very simple:

1 Wash hands in warm water. (This removes any trace of sugar which could distort the reading. It also makes the skin warm and pink so that it is easy to squeeze out a drop of blood.)

2 Choose a finger and squeeze it gently with the other hand forcing the blood to the tip.

3 Prick the side of the finger near the base of the nail lightly with a needle or an automatic pricker. Do not prick the ball which is very sensitive.

4 Squeeze out a drop of blood. (If there is any difficulty about getting a drop, do not poke and prod. Soak the finger in a cup of hand hot water for a few minutes. The blood will spurt out easily after the slightest prick if the finger is very warm.)

5 Turn hand over so that drop hangs down.

6 Drop it neatly onto the end of the plastic strip.

7 Wait for sixty seconds. (It may be longer for higher ranges. Read directions carefully. Different brands may have different times.)

8 Wipe off strip with cotton wool or wash off with water, depending on the brand.

9 Compare colour with the chart or read in reflectance meter.

10 Record result in diary or notebook.

Q. Is this procedure painful or unpleasant in any way?

A. Many children find it preferable to urine testing. With a little practice, most manage to extract the blood drop painlessly. Without exception, they love using the meter and watching the number come up on the display screen. A child who is reluctant to test after realising that it is not painful is probably the child who is apprehensive about the results.

It is important that your child should not associate poor control with being 'naughty'. It is difficult to refrain from an approving word or smile when the test results are good. After all, you are anxious about it and relieved when the test shows that the glucose levels are normal. But every time you say, 'well done' for a good test, your reinforce the idea that somehow poor results are his fault. Perhaps they are. Perhaps he has been careless about his diet or his injections. But generally it is better to encourage him to take an objective view of these tests, regarding them as a guide to management, not a reflection of his conduct. Like the sailor who observes the weather in order to trim his sails, he is not fixing blame for the storm, but must steer a safe course.

Q. Is it necessary to buy the machine to blood test at home?

A. You can buy strips which can be read by eye alone. The end of the strip has a little pad which changes colour according to the amount of glucose in the drop of blood. It is easy to compare the colour to the colour chart on the bottle of strips. If you use the machine, you put the strip into a special place and press a button. The results appear in a display panel which gives you the blood glucose expressed as mmol/l (millimols of glucose per litre of blood). A millimol is a measurement.

Q. Is the machine more accurate than the strips that you read by eye?

A. A study done a few years ago would indicate that they were about equal in accuracy. In both cases, the skill of the user was the most important element. Some people prefer the machine, however, because it is not open to interpretation or influenced by wishful thinking. Cost, however, is a factor for most people.

Q. Are the blood testing strips available under the National Health Service?

A. Not at the moment. It is hoped that this situation will change in the near future. I suggest cutting the strips in half to give you twice as many tests for the money. Some BDA branches buy strips in bulk to sell at a discount to their members. Some clinics give free strips to children who are monitoring at home.

Q. How often should the child do blood tests?

A. Some doctors recommend that the child test once a day. Others prefer that the child select two different days and do four tests on those. Both methods will yield useful information if records are kept.

Q. If a child tests once a day, which times of day are best?

A. Vary the times. Let him test before breakfast on Mondays, before the evening meal on Tuesdays, before bed on Wednesdays, after school on Thursdays, before breakfast on Fridays and before lunch on Saturdays. Take Sundays off. This is only a guide of course. Never arrange tests which will conflict with his social life. He should not be called in from play and forced to test. Never insist. Diabetes is his for life and too much pressure when young could keep him from looking after himself when he is grown.

Q. If he is willing to test regularly at home, does he still have a blood test in the clinic? He dreads this test.

A. The hospital blood test is used for several purposes which you cannot duplicate at home. One important purpose is to measure glycosylated haemoglobin.

Q. What is glycosylated haemoglobin?

A. Red blood cells carry the chemical haemoglobin. Normally, only six per cent of the haemoglobin has glucose molecules attached to it. The red blood cell has a life span of about three months. If the blood glucose has been running higher than usual over this period, a higher percentage of haemoglobin will have glucose attached. The test, called HbAl measures the percentage of haemoglobin with glucose attached. A satisfactory result for a diabetic is nine per cent. If this test is done every three months (which is generally the number of times that the child attends the clinic) you can see how useful it is in determining the level of blood glucose over a long period.

Your child's fear of the blood test is probably because he is afraid of being hurt when the blood is taken. Some clinics rub an analgesic cream on the arm before inserting the needle. This makes the arm less sensitive. Ask in your clinic if such a cream is available.

Q. *Is it possible to be aware of changes in the blood glucose without testing?*

A. When blood glucose falls below normal, the diabetic gets 'hypo' signs. When it rises quite a bit above normal, he feels thirsty, tired and urinates frequently. If, however, the blood glucose is only slightly elevated, there are no obvious symptoms. This is the situation which should be avoided.

Q. *Why is this state particularly dangerous?*

A. If the blood glucose is elevated for long periods of time, the body adjusts. The diabetic feels well, but the persistently high blood sugar can give rise to complications in the future. Also, if he feels well at a higher glucose level than normal, he may feel decidedly unwell and uneasy when better control is instituted and the blood glucose returned to normal. It may take quite a while to get over this feeling. He may resist increasing his insulin because he does not want to feel 'funny'.

Q. *If a child tests his blood regularly, is there a need to do urine tests as well?*

A. Not normally. If, however, he should become ill, it is

important to know whether or not he is producing ketones. The blood tests will not show this. Only the urine tests will pick it up.

Q. Would you recommend the strips or the tablets for urine testing?

A. The strips are simpler and they are easier to keep. Tablets tend to crumble and discolour if they aren't kept absolutely dry. All reagents should be kept dry and the moisture absorbent sachets inside the bottles should not be discarded, but tablets are much harder to store than strips.

Q. Are all brands of strips equally accurate?

A. All the brands which I have used seem to be equally accurate. You should be careful, however, to buy the brand which is meant to do your particular job. If you have a machine, you must buy the sort that goes into the machine. Similarly, if you are reading them by eye, you must buy the correct sort. If your chemist is not familiar with the various brands, he may not be aware of this. At the moment there are two strips available for different machines, Dextrostix, made by Ames and BM strips made by Boelringer Mannheim. Certain machines take one strip, others take the other one. It is important to buy the correct strip for your machine. This information is contained in the literature which comes with the meter. Do not use Dextrostix unless you have a meter. Reading it by eye is extremely difficult.

BM strips are designed to be read either in a meter or by eye. Only certain meters take them however. Another strip, Visidex, is meant for eye reading alone. Visidex is particularly easy to read by eye because it has two colour patches, both yellow. The top patch turns green and the bottom patch turns orange. The bottom patch, however, will not change at all unless the glucose levels are higher than normal. Therefore, you can tell at a glance whether or not you are too high. If the bottom patch remains yellow, you can be certain that the glucose is not elevated.

Q. Are these strips expensive?

A. Visidex is packed in bottles of fifty. If you cut them in half, you can get 100 tests out of a bottle. That costs about 10p per test. If you test six times a week (give him Sundays off), it will cost 60p, half the price of a packet of cigarettes. BM strips come in cans of twenty-five. Similarly, cutting them in half, you get fifty tests for about 12p a test. Dextrostix costs a bit less, about 7p or 8p a test but then you have to have a machine to read them in. Some BDA Branches raise money and buy machines for distribution to children. The Isle of Wight and Enniskillen in Northern Ireland have provided machines for every diabetic child known to them who wants one. Other branches may do the same thing. These groups raise money from the public for this purpose. If you join a self-help group, you might suggest a similar project. Working on ideas like this is a great source of comfort to many parents. It is an opportunity to fight back, a way to help your child and others like him. It can be extremely satisfying.

Q. Why aren't blood testing strips provided by the National Health Service if urine testing strips are?

A. That is a question which you should direct to your MP. I don't know. The only explanation I can think of is that these strips are new and it will take time until their use can be justified for inclusion on the drug tariff.

Q. Is the cost of the strips justified?

A. Absolutely. It is far easier to keep diabetes under control if you can determine with some accuracy the amount of glucose in the blood at any one time. With urine testing alone, the glucose levels that you are observing may not be a true indication of the actual levels in the body. The urine may have been in the bladder for a long time. It is not easy, using urine tests as the only guide, to adjust the insulin dose.

Q. What do you do if you find that there is a high glucose reading before breakfast?

A. If the child is on a combination of clear and cloudy insulin, you increase the cloudy insulin in the *evening* dose. This covers the night-time. Wait then until the next morning. Test again, if it is lower, you have done the right thing. If, however, it is higher and the child complains of a headache, another explanation must be considered. If the evening dose of insulin were too *high* rather than too low, the blood glucose may have gone quite low in the night. This may have gone unnoticed during sleep. The body, however, to protect itself from a hypo, may have released into the bloodstream the extra glucose which is stored in the liver. The blood test in the morning may reflect this.

Q. *Suppose the next morning's reading is lower but still not normal. What do you do then?*

A. Increase the cloudy insulin again.

Q. *How many extra units should you give?*

A. Ask your doctor. There is a great variation in reactions. If you cannot get his advice, increase cautiously one unit per day until you get a satisfactory level in the morning.

Q. *What should you do if the morning's reading is even higher than before you increased the insulin?*

A. Decrease the insulin. If you want to be absolutely positive that you are doing the right thing, test his blood at 2 or 3am. If it is lower than normal then, you should decrease the evening dose.

Q. *Suppose that the child is taking only one injection a day in the morning. It isn't possible to lower the evening dose then so what do you do?*

A. Increase the clear insulin in the morning to lower the blood glucose at once. If you find, however, that he is then going low mid-morning, you could try increasing the circulation instead of increasing the dose. Rub the injection site for five minutes or warm it gently. This will cause the insulin to circulate quicker and bring the glucose levels down without causing a hypo reaction later. If you find that the morning readings are consistently high, you should tell your doctor. It may be that he will recommend a change to a two injection routine in order to improve control.

Q. What do you do if the morning glucose reading is below normal?

A. Lower the evening dose of cloudy insulin if he is on two injections. Solve the immediate problem by giving a glass of orange juice or other quickly-absorbed sugar right away.

Q. Before the injection?

A. Yes. You want to raise the glucose levels before the next dose of insulin takes effect.

Q. What do you do if this problem persists?

A. Tell your doctor. He may want to review the dosage and perhaps make some changes.

Q. How do you treat a high glucose reading before lunch?

A. Increase the morning dose of clear insulin.

Q. What about a low reading before lunch?

A. Reduce the morning dose of clear insulin. Give sugar right away.

Q. What do you do if there is a high reading before the evening meal?

A. Increase the morning dose of cloudy insulin. Also, increase the circulation of the evening injection to solve the immediate problem.

Q. What do you do if there is a hypo before the evening meal?

A. Give sugar. Decrease dose of morning cloudy insulin. If this persists, it might be necessary to move the meal to an earlier time.

Q. How do you treat a high reading before going to bed?

A. Increase the evening dose of clear insulin.

Q. What do you do if the child has a hypo before going to bed?

A. Give sugar. Reduce evening dose of clear insulin.

Q. I know some parents who were warned in hospital never to change their child's insulin dose. What do you advise in that situation?

A. That is very difficult. It is not possible to get good diabetic control if you cannot vary the insulin dose to keep the blood glucose normal. There is certainly not much sense in testing the child's blood or urine for glucose if there is nothing that you can do about it. I think that the best thing to do in those circumstances is to request an interview with the doctor and ask him why he has prohibited changing the dose. Perhaps if he can see that you have a fair understanding of diabetic control, he might feel more confident about allowing changes. I was once at a conference for parents of diabetic children when this question came up. A woman asked it of the distinguished paediatrician who was addressing the meeting, a man with many years of experience as the head of a large clinic and the author of several books on diabetes. His reply was short. I remember it well. 'If your consultant will not allow you to change your child's insulin, change your consultant.'

Q. Is there any other way of controlling the diabetes other than increasing or decreasing insulin?

A. One useful and simple trick is to use time to your benefit. If the reading is slightly too high, give the injection an hour before the meal instead of half an hour before it. That way, the insulin has a chance to act more strongly before more food is taken in.

Q. Normally, what should the time lag be between the injection and the meal?

A. Aim for thirty minutes. Sometimes it is difficult to do this in the morning when everyone seems to be rushing out to school or work but it will give you better control. It is worthwhile to get up a few minutes earlier and do the test and injection before dressing.

Q. I understand that a reading between 4 and 7 mmol/l is normal, but at what point should I start manipulating the insulin? If it is 8 mmol/l or 9 mmol/l should I add a unit?

A. I shouldn't add any insulin until the reading is more than 10 mmol/l unless otherwise instructed by the doctor. With readings between 7 mmol/l and 10 mmol/l, give the injection earlier, try to increase circulation or even reduce the carbohydrate in the meal by 1 exchange.

Q. *What if it is less than 4 mmol/l?*

A. Low blood glucose is easier to deal with in some ways because there is no time to worry about to do. If a hypo is threatened, you must take action immediately by giving sugar. I should do this if the reading is lower than 3.5 mmol/l or if the child feels hypo symptoms.

Q. *What exactly is a hypo?*

A. Hypoglycaemia, usually referred to by diabetics as a hypo, means low blood glucose. Although the scientific definition of hypoglycaemia is a blood glucose less than 2.2 mmol/l, it is possible to show symptoms at levels both higher and lower than this. These symptoms should not be ignored.

Q. *Does a hypo always have a warning period?*

A. In my experience, hypos can be divided into two sorts, mild and severe. The severity of the episode depends on how quickly the blood glucose drops. If it drops gradually, there are warning signs. He might become weak, sweaty, trembly, sick, irritable, numb around the mouth. His vision may blur; he may complain of a headache or a sore tummy. He may weep, appear confused, act drunk. He will probably be unreasonable. If sugar is given as soon as these symptoms appear, the hypo usually subsides in a short time and the child is normal again. If they are not noticed, of course, the blood glucose will continue to drop and the child could become unconscious. There are some episodes of hypoglycaemia which give no warning. Here the blood sugar drops suddenly and rapidly. The person may become unconscious almost immediately. These are rare in childhood.

Q. What happens if my child has a hypo in the night? Will he become unconscious without anyone noticing?

A. Night-time hypoglycaemia is every parent's nightmare. Indeed it is very frightening, especially at first. The early warning stages pass unnoticed in sleep. The child usually wakens, cries, even screams. He may thrash around in his bed and be completely unreasonable and uncontrollable. It may be impossible to persuade him to eat or drink. It is not likely though, that he will become unconscious. It is more likely that he will waken and cry.

Q. If he refuses to take sugar, how can he be helped?

A. There are several things you can do. Don't offer a sweet drink from a glass. If he is screaming and throwing himself around the bed, it is likely that the drink will get everywhere but inside his mouth. Keep a jar of honey or syrup handy. Rub some inside his mouth. He will swallow it with his saliva. Be careful. He might bite you. He will become completely unreasonable and most likely belligerent. If you have a plastic bottle used to wash off the plastic strips before putting them inside the blood testing machine, you can fill it with a sweet drink. These bottles have a curved spout which can be put inside his mouth. You might manage to squirt in the drink. If this fails to help, you could inject him with glucagon.

Q. What is glucagon?

A. Glucagon is a hormone which has the opposite effect of insulin. It causes the liver to release its store of glucose into the bloodstream.

Q. How do you use it?

A. It is injected much like insulin. The glucagon pack consists of two small glass bottles; one containing a powder, the other sterile water. You take an unused insulin syringe (keep a plastic one for this purpose in the refrigerator with the glucagon), draw up all the sterile water, inject it into the powder and mix by shaking the bottle. Draw the mixture into the syringe and inject into the thigh. You may have to sit on him in order to do this. In ten to twenty minutes the child will come round. Then give a sweet drink followed by small amounts of carbohydrate food given frequently. He may feel sick when the glucose level rises. Coca-Cola allowed to go flat is tolerated better when feeling sick than juice or Lucozade. *If consciousness is not regained within 15 or 20 minutes of giving glucagon, intravenous glucose is required from a doctor.*

Q. *Is glucagon difficult to use?*
A. The greatest difficulty in using glucagon is using it under stress. It is a good idea to practise with an extra packet sometime. Get an out-of-date pack from another parent or from the chemist. Practise opening the bottles and mixing the glucagon. This practise will give you confidence. Don't worry about its use. It is not a drug. It is a hormone and the amount in the bottle is small.

Q. *Where can I get glucagon?*
A. You get it in the chemist's on prescription.

Q. *What do I do if my doctor does not approve of its use?*
A. If your doctor does not want you to use glucagon and you cannot get the child to accept sugar, take him to the nearest hospital.

Q. *What would happen if no one heard his cries?*
A. Probably, he would fall asleep, his glucose levels would rise naturally in response to the hypoglycaemia and he would wake up in the morning with a headache. Most night-time hypos do pass unnoticed. The body has a natural mechanism for coping with low glucose levels. The level of glucagon in the body will rise, triggering the release of glucose from the liver. When you inject artificial glucagon, you are merely speeding up this natural process. You are not giving a drug.

Q. *What is the reason for hypos?*
A. A hypo can occur if the insulin level is not balanced by the carbohydrate intake. If, for example, the child has his usual amount of insulin in the morning but then plays a vigorous

game of football without taking any extra carbohydrate, his blood glucose may drop too low. If a meal or a snack is forgotten, there may be too much insulin in the bloodstream and not enough food for it to work on. *Balance* is the key to diabetic control; balance and regularity.

Q. *What do you mean by 'regularity'?*
A. Diabetic control is much easier if the diabetic rises at the same time every day, takes his meals at the same time every day and goes to bed at the same time every evening. Nothing will throw the diabetes off balance quicker than missed snacks, late meals or staying in bed very late on weekend and holiday mornings.

Q. *If my child has a bad hypo in the night, shall I keep him from school next day?*
A. You will have to judge his state of health in the morning. It is likely that he will not remember the events of the previous night even though the rest of the family are still upset. He may have a headache. His blood sugar will undoubtedly be high. This is only temporary. It will drop later in the day. If he wants to go to school, I would be inclined to let him. I would give him extra carbohydrate to take if he should feel low again. (This is very unlikely but it will make you feel better.) You should ring the school and ask them to let you know if he becomes unwell. (This probably won't happen either but it will make you feel better.) Hypos are much more distressing to the parent than to the child who will not recollect them.

Q. *What can I do to ensure that it will not recur?*
A. Review the events of the previous days in your mind. Were there small signals that you overlooked? Did he have several episodes of mild hypoglycaemia which you counteracted by giving an extra snack or moving up his meal time? Did he eat all his snack on the evening of the hypo? Was it large enough? Did he use up more energy than usual in play that day? Could his insulin be reduced without sending up his blood glucose? If you think it could, try it. Ring the clinic and ask for their advice.

Remember that home blood monitoring is a faithful guide. It is the blood glucose tests which allow you to make an intelligent, informed decision. You should keep in mind, however, the fact that the diabetes will become unstable at times even though you have been doing all the right things. Sometimes the insulin is absorbed more quickly than usual. There is really no way of knowing this. Severe hypos are rare in a child whose diabetes is well controlled.

Q. *Do hypos occur at school?*

A. They can, so the staff should know how to cope. A child who takes the school dinner might encounter a menu he doesn't like. He eats less than usual, plays hard afterwards and the result could be a hypoglycaemic episode in the afternoon. If the early signs are noticed by his friend or the teacher, glucose tablets, sweets or a drink could be given at once avoiding a real medical problem perhaps one in which the child becomes unconscious or has a fit.

Q. *Are fits common during a hypo?*

A. Some children have them if the blood glucose drops suddenly. A fit is very upsetting to the parent but there is no evidence that it does permanent damage to the child. If your child has a fit you should inform the doctor about it and reduce his insulin.

Q. *Are hypos more common at night?*

A. Not necessarily, but everything seems worse in the middle of the night. The parents are not at their best at 3 o'clock in the morning, awakened from sleep, trying to cope with an unreasonable child in a cold house without any warning. Everything seems worse at such a time. Hypos can occur at any time but during the day the child or the parent will usually recognise the warning signals and sugar can be taken immediately to correct the situation.

Q. *How long does it take after sugar is given for the hypo to go away?*

A. In a mild hypo, where warning signs are noted and sugar taken the symptoms will go in about five minutes. A headache may linger though.

Q. *How do you cope with a very young child who cannot recognise the symptoms?*

A. You have to be extremely observant and vigilant in sticking to the diabetic regime. Keeping to exact meal times and snack times will help to keep the diabetes balanced. Keep a watchful eye on him if he should suddenly stop playing and become quiet. Many young children get very pale if their glucose levels fall. Err on the side of caution here. If you think that he may be going hypo, give him a sweet drink immediately. If he recovers himself in a few minutes you will know that you were right. If he continues to act strangely, keep him under observation. With small bodies, things happen quickly. Perhaps he is coming down with an infection. If you are worried, test his blood. You will find this a great source of comfort in times of uncertainty.

Q. *I think that my child's blood glucose is higher on clinic days than on other days. Is this a coincidence?*

A. It is difficult to measure stress but it is common knowledge that stress raises the blood glucose. I don't think that this is a coincidence. This is another reason for testing regularly at home. If a single test performed in the clinic is used as the only guide to insulin dosage, many diabetics would be taking too much insulin.

Q. *Can school pressure raise the glucose?*

A. Any stress can raise the blood glucose. This is part of the body's mechanism for fighting back. Your child, however, should not be encouraged to use his diabetes as an excuse for poor school performance. Missing school days certainly has an effect on performance. You can play a significant role in ensuring that the usual illnesses of childhood do not upset the diabetic control.

Q. *Can a minor illness like a cold upset the diabetes?*

A. Generally, at the first sign of an illness, even a minor one, the blood glucose goes up. Sometimes, even with a minor infection, the glucose rises quite high and ketones may be formed.

Q. Why does this happen?

A. Insulin is a storage hormone. If the body lacks insulin, it cannot store glucose or fat. When fat molecules are broken down (because they cannot be stored) they release ketones into the bloodstream. If the body is overwhelmed by ketones, serious illness, even death can result. When your child first developed diabetes, he was producing ketones. The symptoms of ketone production are abdominal pain, vomitting, deep sighing breathing and eventually coma. He was also very thirsty, passed large amounts of urine, perhaps was very tired and lethargic. These are symptoms of a high blood glucose. The presence of ketones is an indication that insulin is urgently required.

Q. How do you know when ketones are present?

A. They are detectable in the urine. At the first sign of illness, test the urine for ketones using reagent strips or tablets. Even if the test is negative, continue to test the urine several times a day until the illness has passed. Sometimes, in their enthusiasm for blood testing, people forget that urine testing still has a part to play in diabetic control.

Q. What should be done if ketones are present?

A. Give more insulin.

Q. How much more?

A. Ring the clinic if you can. If you cannot get any medical advice, increase by 2 units of clear insulin and test often to see whether this is enough. If the child is feverish you may need to give more clear insulin.

Q. What happens if the child cannot eat enough food to cope with the increased insulin?

A. Give him light foods which are tolerated easily when ill; jellies, fruit juice, milk with honey or syrup, Coca-Cola, lemonade, tea with sugar, Ribena, Lucozade, apple purée, ice-cream, etc.

Q. *What should be done if he cannot take enough to make up the right amount of carbohydrate for a meal?*

A. Don't worry about making up enough for a meal. Offer these foods often. Let him take one portion every hour if that is all he can tolerate.

Q. *What shall I do if he refuses all food or is sick?*

A. If he will not or cannot eat or drink consider it an emergency. You need medical help. If you cannot get any advice, take him to the Casualty Department of the nearest hospital, especially if he is being sick. Do not delay. A diabetic who is manufacturing ketones and who is vomiting needs professional medical treatment.

Q. *Shall I reduce or stop his insulin if he is vomiting?*

A. No. *Never stop the insulin.* An insulin-dependent diabetic needs insulin every day. More insulin may be needed during his illness. The answer to this question lies in the results of the urine tests. If they show glucose and ketones, he needs more insulin. The urine tests are your best guide during illness. Even if you are blood testing regularly, *return to urine testing during illness.*

Q. *Is it likely that my child will be hospitalized more often now that he is a diabetic?*

A. No, not at all. By observing a few simple rules, the diabetic child can be looked after at home in the same way as the non-diabetic child. The important points to remember are:
1 Act quickly. Do not wait to see how things develop. Most infections are more easily treated in the early stages.
2 More, not less insulin is required during illness.
3 Test the urine for glucose and ketones several times a day.
4 Test the blood glucose several times a day.
5 Switch to a light diet even though these sugary foods are generally avoided.

Q. *Now that my child has become diabetic, will he be ill more often?*

A. There is no evidence to show that he will be ill more often.

What will happen, however, is that the diabetes will require more attention during periods of illness because the blood glucose will rise and ketones may be formed. You will find that you will be able to keep the diabetes under control by increasing the insulin.

Q. Will the diabetes affect other aspects of health care like teeth?

A. Diabetes does not affect the teeth but neglected teeth can cause ill health. All children should attend the dentist regularly. Try to keep your child's schedule in mind when arranging for dental work to be done. Make sure that it doesn't interfere with his lunch or snack time. If a dental appointment is scheduled just before lunch and the child has to wait for a long time for his turn, his blood glucose might drop below normal. If he has to wait for a long time after treatment before he can eat, it could cause a problem. Tell the dentist that he is a diabetic and must have his meals on time. Also, if he has to have a tooth extracted or any other work done under a general anaesthetic, this must be done in hospital. The dentist must confer with the doctor who is treating the diabetes before any such dental work is undertaken.

Q. Can the diabetic child have a local anaesthetic for dental treatment?

A. He can have an injection of novocaine. For any other anaesthetic (gas, for example) the dentist should confer with the doctor in charge.

Q. Can the diabetic child take the same medicine as the non-diabetic? I am thinking of the sugary solutions in which children's antibiotics are mixed and also about cough syrups.

A. The most urgent requirement of the ill diabetic is to get well. If there is an alternative to sugary medicines, your doctor can prescribe them. If not, it is more important to clear the infection than to count the carbohydrates. A teaspoon of a child's antibiotic only contains 5 grams of carbohydrate anyway. If the child needs an antibiotic, it is likely that he has a fever, his blood glucose is elevated and he is producing ketones as well. He will, therefore, be taking extra insulin that day which will cover the sugar in the medicine.

Q. I have heard that girls can get an itchy discharge from the vagina when they are diabetic. Is this common and what causes it?

A. This condition is not uncommon when the diabetes is first discovered. It is called thrush and is caused by organisms which thrive in a sugary environment. It is not serious and will generally clear up when the blood glucose is lowered. If it is bothersome, the doctor can prescribe a cream. Sometimes this condition recurs after insulin therapy is established. It is a sign that the blood glucose is too high. More frequent blood tests will guide you in adjusting the insulin to keep the glucose levels near normal.

Q. Can boys get a similar infection?

A. They can but it is less common. The end of the penis can become sore and the foreskin thickened. This too is caused by high concentrations of sugar. Keeping the urine free from glucose will clear it up. Keeping the diabetes under control will keep the genital area free from these infections.

Q. My child complains sometimes of blurred vision. What is the cause of this?

A. Changes in the levels of blood glucose, either rising or falling, can cause blurred vision. This is not a serious condition. It is usually temporary but it is one which should be reported to your doctor. Check the glucose levels often by testing blood or urine and try to bring the diabetes under steadier control.

Q. I know that diabetes can cause blindness. Does this happen to children?

A. The conditions which lead to blindness take many years to develop. The tiny blood vessels in the retina at the back of the eye can be damaged or cataracts may develop affecting vision. It occurs in a mild degree in many diabetic adults but is serious in only a few.

Q. Can this be treated?

A. Retinal damage can be treated most successfully provided that it is treated in the early stages. It can be treated by laser therapy by a process called photocoagulation. This is not a surgical procedure. Cataracts can also be removed. Your diabetic clinic will arrange for regular eye examinations for your child. Problems are more likely after years of poor control. The best prevention is to keep the blood glucose as near normal as you can.

Q. What about other complications?

A. The most common complications of diabetes are retinopathy (eye) nephropathy (kidney) and neuropathy (nerve). It is possible that they are the consequences of long term abnormalities in blood glucose levels. There is evidence to show that diabetics who are well controlled from the onset of the disease will be less likely to develop these complications. It is very important that you teach your child responsible attitudes towards his diabetes. He should regard the clinic as a helpful place, the diagnostic tests as preventative rather than unpleasant and the manipulation of his insulin to achieve normal glucose levels as part of life.

7

Travelling

Q. When travelling abroad, is it wise to carry an identifying letter in the language of the country in case of illness?

A. Yes. The BDA have cards in several languages for this purpose. They can be carried in handbags or pockets. In addition, it is a good idea to have a letter to be produced at the Customs desk if questioned about the large number of syringes, insulin bottles, needles, etc. in your bag. There is always the danger that this equipment may be confused with the supplies of drug addicts. A letter from your doctor on hospital stationery with a translation below the English text is very useful.

Q. Where can I get such a letter?

A. Your doctor can provide the English text, of course. A travel agent might be able to suggest a translator. Perhaps a foreign student or shopkeeper can help. If you cannot find anyone, contact the nearest college or university where courses are offered in the language you require. As a last resort, you can write to the consulate or embassy of the country you propose to visit. Allow plenty of time for a reply.

Q. What extra equipment do I need to carry for my child when travelling?

A. Take plenty of everything. Remember that insulin strengths on the Continent are different from those in the UK, Ireland, US, Canada and Australia. If you need to buy extra insulin on the Continent, you will have to buy it in 40 or 80 strengths and estimate the proper dosage. Why give yourself that worry! Anticipate breaking or losing a few bottles and bring plenty of extras. Use disposable syringes for travelling even if you use a glass syringe at home. Even if you have a blood testing meter, you will probably find it handier to carry the strips you read by eye while travelling. Pack all your equipment into two bags, each set complete down to the last detail. Keep one set on your person at all times. That way, you can be certain that missing baggage will not throw you into a tizz and spoil your holiday. Naturally, you will not pack insulin into a bag which will be stored in the baggage compartment of an aircraft because of the danger of freezing. Keep the insulin in your hand luggage on the plane.

Q. Will going through the X-ray machines at the airport affect the insulin?

A. No.

Q. Will the insulin keep in a hot climate?

A. According to the manufacturers, it will keep stable in temperatures up to 25°C for a month. Try, however, to keep it as cool as possible. If there is no fridge or ice box available to you, you can bring an insulated picnic bag from home. You can probably find a way of getting ice or freezing sachets for the bag. If you have no other way of keeping it cool, wrap the bottles in wet cloth. Keep the cloth wet all the time. The constant evaporation of the water will keep the bottle cool in the same way that panting keeps a dog cool. Don't leave insulin in the glove compartment or boot of the car as these areas heat up quickly in the sun.

Q. Can you give me a check list for travelling?

A.
● Twice as much insulin as you think you will need
● Glucagon
● Extra syringes and needles
● Urine testing strips for glucose and ketones
● Blood testing strips
● Lancet for pricking fingers
● Mediswabs
● Injector if needed (an extra if possible)
● ID cards and letter if travelling abroad
● Inside EEC, form E111 from DHSS
● Outside EEC, health insurance
● ID bracelet or necklace
● Food and drink

Q. *How does one cope with flying through time zones?*

A. Flying from East to West (London to New York for example), the day will be five hours longer. The diabetic will need an extra injection of cloudy insulin to cope with a bedtime which will be at two or three in the morning and extra meals. This injection should be done before bedtime. Your doctor will advise the amount.

Flying West to East (New York to London for example), the day will be five hours shorter. The diabetic should reduce his insulin before the evening meal and take an extra injection of long acting insulin before bed. Again, your doctor will advise the amount required.

8

Diabetes in Adolescents and Young Adults

Q. Is diabetes more difficult in adolescence?

A. Everything seems to be more difficult in adolescence. It is hard for the adolescent to cope with all the strange and exciting changes that are happening to his body. It may make him moody and hard to live with. If he has to cope with diabetes as well, it imposes a great strain. I have seen many a cheerful, compliant diabetic child who has been keeping to his food plan, testing his blood at home, and presenting a picture of cooperation in the clinic change almost overnight into a sullen, uncooperative adolescent, snapping at his mother, avoiding the doctor's eye, forgetting his record book and refusing to see the dietician. This is all quite normal. There is no need for parents to be embarrassed at the attitude of this newly grown monster. In a few years, she or he will revert to the pleasant cooperative person who was hiding inside that teenage dragon.

Q. Can anything be done to ease the child through this period?

A. One idea which might be helpful to parents of the newly diagnosed diabetic is to be sure to let the diabetes be *his* not yours. If you take over the control completely, when it comes time to rebel against your authority, he will rebel against the diabetes as well. No matter how young the child, it is important to handle things as soon as he is able. Even if you can do it better or quicker, so long as he is capable of doing it safely, he should be allowed. It is your role as parent to teach him to look after himself, not do everything for him.

Even young children can get their own snacks, keep their diabetic kit in order, enter blood and urine tests results in the diary or notebook, and learn the carbohydrate value of foods. A school-age child can become quite expert. He should be encouraged to learn about his diabetes. There are several excellent booklets written for children which can probably be found in your clinic or your local BDA Branch. When he has learned a little, he should be consulted when his regime has to be changed. It is quite in order for the parent to say, 'You have had two hypos recently; what do you think we should do to prevent any more?' *Balance* has articles and stories for children. Sometimes they solicit letters and stories or drawings from them too. Encourage your child to participate. If you join the local Branch, he can get pleasure from helping to raise money for diabetic research. Good attitudes developed in childhood will make adolescence less painful.

Q. Does sleeping late in the morning on weekends and holidays affect control?

A. Diabetes is thrown off balance by missed snacks, late meals and delayed injections. This can be a problem in adolescence. I think that the best plan is to compromise a bit. Allow an extra hour on a weekend morning. If your child wants to have more than an extra hour in bed (and who doesn't?), he will have to compromise a little too. Let him get up, do his injection, fix himself a breakfast tray and take it back to his room. After he has eaten his breakfast, he can lounge about in his room, even go back to sleep if he likes and still not disturb his diabetic control.

Q. Is control upset during adolescence due to physical changes in the child?

A. Yes. Many girls will find that diabetic control becomes erratic during the menstrual period. Extra blood tests on those days is a good idea so that insulin needs can be responded to. Stress is a factor in control as well. In periods of stress the blood sugar rises. Hyperglycaemia (high blood glucose; see Appendix 3 on p 111 for a discussion of symptoms and treatment) may result. Since adolescence is a stressful time, episodes of hyperglycaemia may be more frequent than in childhood. This can be coped with by increasing the insulin. The important thing to remember about adolescence is that it isn't permanent. Try to keep your sense of humour intact even if your child appears to have mislaid his.

Q. Will diabetes affect the sex life of the young adult?
A. I don't see any reason why it should. As regards sexuality, young diabetics are no different from young non-diabetics.

Q. What about impotency? I have heard that diabetes can cause impotency in men.
A. Impotency can be a problem for men who have diabetic neuropathy of long standing. I have never heard of a young diabetic male becoming impotent.

Q. Can diabetes affect menstruation?
A. The onset of menstruation is sometimes delayed in the diabetic girl. Once menstruation begins, there should be no special problems due to the diabetes. The possible delay in beginning menstruation should be explained to the diabetic girl. Girls of this age look forward eagerly to their first menstrual period. It can be very disappointing to a young girl to feel that she is left behind when all her friends are becoming young women. She should be reassured that her time will come even if it is postponed somewhat. In this area too, good control plays a part.

Q. Are there other problems associated with growth and sexual development?
A. It is rare today for diabetes to affect growth unless control has been very poor in the early years. Your child will be weighed and measured at every clinic visit and his growth carefully noted. If you are anxious on this point, discuss it with your doctor. Some parents are so worried about taking up the doctor's time that they feel timid about asking questions. Sometimes the doctor has more patients to see than he can manage in the allotted time; he looks rushed and doesn't encourage conversation. If this is the situation in your clinic, write down your questions at home when you are

relaxed. That way the doctor's attention can be directed to the important issues which worry you without any time consuming preliminaries.

Q. Can a diabetic use the pill?

A. She can. Most doctors agree that there is no increased risk to diabetics in using any one type of birth control; the pill, the coil, the sheath, etc. are all acceptable.

What should be emphasised to girls is that it is very important that the blood glucose be normal *before* conception as well as during pregnancy. *Planning* is essential to the diabetic pregnancy and an early consultation with the doctor is advised. I think that pregnancy will be one area where the insulin pump will be of great value.

Q. Is pregnancy difficult or dangerous for diabetics?

A. The management of the diabetic pregnancy has improved enormously over the years. Today, specialist antenatal clinics for diabetics have demonstrated that on a regime of three or four injections a day, the diabetic can keep her glucose levels normal during pregnancy.

Q. Can she have a normal delivery?

A. More diabetic women are having normal deliveries than ever before. Diabetics used to produce very large babies which made caesarian sections almost obligatory. With better control during pregnancy, babies can be kept to normal size.

Q. What caused these babies to be so large?

A. High maternal blood glucose during pregnancy caused the babies to gain more weight than normal. That is one reason why it is essential to maintain normal glucose levels during pregnancy.

Q. Is this difficult?

A. Women are motivated during pregnancy to look after themselves better. Increasing the number of injections and doing several blood tests a day can keep the blood glucose levels normal. Also, during pregnancy, hormonal changes make diabetic control easier. If normal glucose levels are maintained during pregnancy (and they can be) the outcome of the pregnancy should be no different than if the woman were not diabetic.

Q. Can the diabetic mother breastfeed her baby?
A. There is no reason why the diabetic mother should not breastfeed her baby. She may have to increase the number of calories she eats and therefore a slight increase in insulin may be necessary too. After delivery, however, frequent changes of insulin are necessary to adjust to the non-pregnant state. Hormonal changes in the first few days after the birth will result in changes in insulin requirements.

Q. Will the pregnant diabetic be admitted to hospital early?
A. Possibly she will be admitted a few weeks before the baby is due to keep perfect control in the last weeks of pregnancy. Some antenatal clincs, though, allow pregnant diabetics to wait until full term at home if there are no problems.

Q. Will the baby be induced early?
A. When babies were larger than normal, it was the custom to deliver diabetics before full term. Today, however, with perfect control possible, the situation is different. If there is a choice of medical care available during pregnancy, it is a good idea to find a specialized diabetic antenatal clinic where the most modern methods are used.

Q. Is there a chance that the baby will be diabetic?
A. The chance is very small. It should not be a deterrent to having a family.

Q. Can a diabetic have an abortion?
A. Diabetics can have abortions just like non-diabetics. It is very important, though, that any operation requiring a general anaesthetic be performed in hospital so that the staff are aware that the patient is an insulin-dependent diabetic. Abortion, however, is traumatic for everyone. This is a situation which is far better avoided. A girl's best friend in

DIABETES IN ADOLESCENTS AND YOUNG ADULTS

these matters should be her mother. If mothers strive to keep the channels of communication open between them and their adolescent daughters, it is less likely that girls will become pregnant out of ignorance or spite. Sometimes, young pregnant girls are secretly pleased by the prospect of thwarting domineering parents or by the thought of having someone who will be helpless and dependent on them. Adolescence is a time of expansion and experimentation but it is also a time when the security of childhood is still required. Give your child room to try new ideas and independence but always ensure that the way back to you is left open. The young diabetic needs this reassurance even more because for him the road to independence is more precarious.

Q. *Would it be better for diabetic students to attend college near home rather than go far away where they would be in complete control of their condition without any help?*

A. If your child has been taught how to look after himself from the time that he is first diagnosed, he should be quite able to care for himself by the time he reaches college age. The decision about which university or college to go to is a scholastic not a medical decision. It may be that only a particular institution offers the course he wants. He may be looking forward (he *should* be looking forward) to an opportunity to live in a new place, make new friends and be more independent. His diabetes should not rob him of that chance. If it does, he is very likely to rebel against it. Besides, your child will not be in complete control of his condition. He will have friends who will help him. He will also have medical help near the college. Your child should attend a clinic nearby so that his medical records will be accessible in case of need. He should find a friend who can learn about diabetes and help him.

Q. *Should he have a room mate?*

A. If he likes the idea of sharing a room, yes. That would be a good way of ensuring that someone would always be aware if he had a problem like a night-time hypo. If, however, he prefers to room alone, he might be able to ask a neighbour to keep an eye on him. If he is mature enough to live away from home he must be mature enough to ask for this kind of assistance without embarrassment.

Q. Is alcohol a problem to a diabetic?

A. Although many diabetics drink alcohol, drinking can be a problem. There are many reasons for this. One reason is that alcohol can bring on a hypo. If a diabetic becomes hypo after alcohol, it will appear to others (perhaps the police) that he is drunk and disorderly. His diabetes may not be apparent even if he has a card in his pocket or an ID bracelet around his wrist. He may be put somewhere to 'sleep it off', and he may go into a coma. Tragedy could be the result. Diabetics should only drink alcohol with food. The carbohydrate in the drink should never be used in exchange for carbohydrate food. Drinking on an empty stomach should be avoided. It can have disastrous effects by lowering the blood glucose quickly. Food should be eaten before any alcohol is taken.

Q. What about diabetic beer?

A. Diabetic beer contains less carbohydrate than other beers, just as much or more alcohol and just as many calories.

Q. What drink is the safest?

A. Avoid drinks which are very sweet like fortified wines and spirits mixed with lemonade, tonic or coke. Dry wines, sherries and spirits with low calorie mixers are probably best.

Q. What advice can you give to a young person wishing to go out with friends to a pub?

A. 1 Let your friends know that you are diabetic and exactly what this means as regards alcohol.

2 Eat a good meal before you go.

3 Drink moderately. One or two beers should be enough.

4 Eat something with the drinks. A bag of crisps would help.

5 Don't miss any meals or snacks while you are in the pub.

6 If the drinking session goes on for a long time and you feel that you cannot excuse yourself, switch to a sugarless soft drink. If the others are drinking gin, whisky or rum, no one will notice that your drink is a mixer only. If they are drinking pints of beer or stout, sip yours slowly.

Try to remember that it isn't adult to make yourself ill. It's stupid.

Q. What shall I do if my adolescent comes home drunk?
A. Make sure that he isn't hypo. Do a blood test. If his glucose is normal, let him sleep for a while. If it is low, try to get him to take some sugar. Treat it as any other hypo.

Q. Is it dangerous for diabetics to take drugs?
A. Yes, very dangerous. The most important element in good diabetic control are balance and regularity. Drug-taking is a major disturbance to the body. Parents cannot be too emphatic in explaining this to their children. Drug abuse is absolutely incompatible and may even be life threatening to the diabetic.

Q. Is this true for cannabis as well as the harder drugs?
A. Yes. Even with a drug which may be only mildly halluci-natory, a diabetic may forget to eat his meals or take his injections because of the euphoria. Warning symptoms of a hypo may go unnoticed for the same reason.

Q. What should a parent do if he or she suspects that the diabetic child is experimenting with hard drugs?
A. Contact your diabetic clinic and discuss the problem with the staff. It may be necessary to inform the authorities. Parents cannot cope with this problem themselves. It requires expert handling.

Q. How can parents convince an adolescent whose friends use drugs that he must not indulge?
A. An adolescent is old enough to live with the knowledge that diabetes is a potentially fatal disease. Only careful manage-ment on his part is keeping him alive. If he opts out of this

management, he will not survive. Drug taking is opting out. It is my experience that most young people are frightened by the drug scene and will seize on an excuse to reject it if that excuse is acceptable to their friends. Diabetes must be seen to be an acceptable excuse. Perhaps a family friend, doctor or some other person, an older diabetic maybe, could help to convince your child that it is so. At this sensitive age, an adolescent may accept advice more easily from someone outside the family. Try to find someone whom he particularly admires and ask that person to talk to him.

Q. Should diabetics smoke?
A. No. Diabetes is a risk factor in the development of heart disease. Smoking is also a risk factor. The combination could be significant. Smoking also inhibits the absorption of insulin.

Q. How can I discourage my child from smoking when other members of the family smoke?
A. You can't. Children tend to do what we do rather than what we say. If you want to ensure that your diabetic child does not smoke, you'll probably have to stop smoking yourself.

Q. Is it all right for diabetics to attend discos and parties which go on for long periods and where alcohol is served?
A. By disco-going age your child should be able to take charge of his diabetes himself. It is really up to him to demonstrate that he knows how to cope with late hours, frantic activity and excitement. Disco dancing uses up a lot of energy and probably requires extra carbohydrate. This would be readily available in the form of soft drinks and snacks. Excess alcohol can be refused and an occasional late night will not upset the diabetic control. Denying him permission to do what his friends are allowed to do will upset his control more.

In this situation, as in many others in childhood and adolescence, the child's best friend can be a great help. If the friend can be stimulated to take an interest in diabetes, perhaps given books to read if that is appropriate or even invited to accompany the diabetic child on various outings sponsored by the BDA, that can be a great advantage to the family. I know one family where the diabetic child's best friend can fill the syringe, do blood tests, count carbohydrate exchanges and recognise the signs of impeding hypo-glycaemia. With her friend, the diabetic child has success-fully gone on camping trips for a week at a time, hiked long distances and competed in swimming competitions far from home.

Q. How old should the diabetic child be before being allowed away from home?

A. No matter what the child's age, it is a good idea to let the first period away from home after diagnosis be one in which the diabetes can be looked after by trained staff. A BDA holiday camp is ideal for this purpose. Children from six or seven up to late teens can be accommodated. Children can participate in all sorts of social and athletic activities confident that help is at hand if required. The camp also gives the newly-diagnosed diabetic the opportunity to learn more about his diabetes. He is in an environment in which he is no different from any other child. This helps most children to come to terms with the condition. It also gives parents a much needed break, especially needed soon after diagnosis when life is particularly stressful and bewildering.

Q. Should the diabetic adolescent be allowed to drive a car?

A. Driving is very important in our culture. It is regarded by many youngsters as a coming-of-age ceremony, a rite of passage from childhood to adult life. Refusing him per-mission to drive will only cause him to feel deprived and resentful. I should allow it provided that he can demonstrate to your complete satisfaction that he is looking after himself responsibly. He must, therefore, be willing to test his blood each time he gets behind the wheel and take appropriate food or drink if his blood glucose is below 5 mml/l. Low blood glucose will impede his reactions and possibly cause an accident.

Q. Can a diabetic get car insurance?

A. Yes, but he might have to pay a bit extra. The BDA are very helpful in recommending insurance companies which issue policies to diabetics. If you write or ring them, they can give you this information.

Q. Does he have to inform the licensing authorities that he is diabetic?

A. Yes. There is a question on the licence application about it. It is very important that he answer this question truthfully. If he does not admit his diabetes on the form, his insurance will not be valid and should he have an accident, even one completely unconnected with his diabetes or one in which he is completely blameless, his insurance cover will be void.

Q. Will he have to present medical evidence to get his licence?

A. Generally, if a person is an insulin-dependent diabetic, he must have a letter from his doctor saying that the diabetes is well controlled.

Q. What about driving a motor bike?

A. Much as parents might shrink from the thought of this activity with all its attendant dangers, the same principle must prevail. If he would be allowed to do this as a non-diabetic, his diabetes must not be allowed to stand in the way. If he is responsible enough to do frequent blood tests and not drive if his blood glucose is below 5 mml/l, carry sugar with him on his person, stop and take sugar at the first sign of a hypo, abstain from alcohol when on the bike, carry an ID card or wear identifying jewellery, then permission should be given or withheld on the same grounds that it would be if he were not diabetic.

Q. Does the diabetes have to be declared to the licensing authorities for a motor bike licence?

A. If there is a question on the application form about disqualifying diseases, he must admit the diabetes. A letter from the doctor, however, will probably satisfy the authorities.

Q. I have heard that family doctors charge large sums for this letter. Is that true?

A. It depends entirely on the doctor. The general practitioner is not an employee of the National Health Service. He is a private contractor. If you think that his fee is unreasonable, ask the consultant in the diabetic clinic to do it. Hospital doctors are employees of the NHS and can provide such letters without charge.

Q. Are there any jobs barred to diabetics?

A. Yes, a diabetic will not be accepted in the Armed Forces, Police or Fire Service or for training as a long distance lorry driver or driver of a public vehicle such as bus, train or airline pilot. It would be wiser for them to have an occupation which kept their feet on the ground. This rules out being a steeple jack. They can do most other types of work. Many diabetics are doctors, nurses, teachers, secretaries, farmers, actors, professional athletes, etc. There is a wide realm of occupations open to diabetics and your youngster should never feel that diabetes has seriously limited his choice of careers.

9

The Last Question

Q. What do you do if an injection is forgotten? How quickly do things happen?

A. If your child forgets his injection, he will probably begin to feel unwell after a few hours. His blood glucose will rise rapidly. But whatever you do, *don't panic*. You can give the missing injection and things will settle down in a few hours. If he isn't sure as to whether or not he did his injection, test his blood. If he didn't take the insulin, his blood glucose will be high. Give a small injection of clear acting insulin and test him again in a few hours. If glucose levels have returned to normal, forget the incident. If they are still very high, give another small injection. Give him his meals at the usual time. By the time his next injection time comes around, he will have returned to normal.

Appendices

Appendix 1

Injection Sites

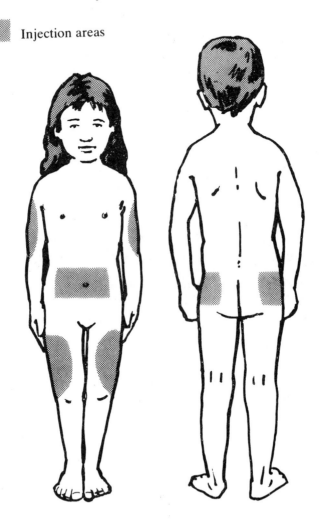

Injection areas

Appendix 2

Hypoglycaemia (low blood glucose)

Symptoms
- weakness
- sweating
- trembling
- sickness
- irritability
- weeping
- blurring of vision
- seeing double
- headache
- sore tummy
- confusion
- appears drunk

What to do at first
- drink Ribena, Lucozade, Coca-Cola, juice, sweet tea, etc.
- eat sweets, glucose tablets (2–4), sugar lumps

What to do next
- take snack of milk and biscuits or sandwich eat meal if almost meal time

What to do if first remedies fail or if child is unconscious
- rub inside of mouth with honey or syrup
- inject glucagon
- take child to Casualty Ward of nearest hospital

Hyperglycaemia (high blood glucose)

Symptoms
- thirst
- frequent passing of urine
- high blood sugars
- urine tests show 2% (darkest colour) for 3 days

What to do
- increase insulin
- if caused by infection, get medical help for illness
- if caused by too much carbohydrate, check list
- if symptoms persist, call the doctor

Diabetic ketoacidosis

(very high blood glucose with ketones)

Symptoms
- increasing thirst
- frequent passing of urine
- urine tests show 2% (darkest colour) for more than 2 tests in the day
- urine tests show ketones for more than 2 tests in the day
- sickness or vomiting
- tummy pain
- cold and dry skin
- deep breathing

What to do
Do not delay in obtaining medical help. Ring your doctor. If you cannot get medical help at home, take the child to the Casualty Ward of the nearest hospital. You cannot look after ketoacidosis at home.

Useful items

Items available under the National Health Service in 1986

insulin
glass syringe
needles
cotton wool
industrial spirit
cotton swabs
glucagon
tablets and strips for urine tests
test tubes
droppers

Items which must be purchased

plastic syringes
strips for blood testing
some strips for ketones
spirit case for glass syringe
injection aids
blood testing monitor
finger pricker

Items available to BDA members

Balance
discounts through the branch on bulk
items like blood testing strips
posters
books, films, videos available for purchase at reasonable prices

Items available free on request from pharmaceutical companies

booklets, leaflets, posters about diabetes
tape-slide programmes available to groups

Items available from BDA to groups

video films
16mm films

Some Books about Diabetes

Dr James Anderson, *Diabetes* (Martin Dunitz)

Dr Arnold Bloom, *Diabetes Explained* (MTP Press Ltd.)

British Diabetic Association, *Cooking the New Diabetic Way* (Ward Lock Ltd.)

British Diabetic Association, *Countdown*

British Diabetic Association, *The Diabetics Handbook* (Jaguar Press Ltd.)

Drs Ireland, Thomson and Williamson, *Diabetes Today* (HM & M)

Dr Jim Mann, *The Diabetics' Diet Book* (Martin Dunitz)

Index